FAMILY DOCTORS AND ECONOMIC INCENTIVES

For David, Helen, Kate and Matthew

Family Doctors and Economic Incentives

Nick Bosanquet
Brenda Leese

Centre for Health Economics
University of York

Dartmouth

Published by

Dartmouth Publishing Company,
Gower House, Croft Road, Aldershot,
Hants. GU11 3HR, England

Gower Publishing Company
Old Post Road, Brookfield, Vermont 05036
USA

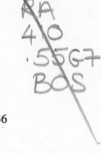

British Library Cataloguing in Pulication Data
Bosanquet, Nicholas.
Family doctors and economic incentives.
1. Great Britain. Medicine. Economic aspects
I. Title II. Leese, Brenda
338.4'761'0941

Printed by Athenæum Press
Newcastle upon Tyne

ISBN 1 85521 009 6

Contents

Contents

Acknowledgements

This study has been assisted by a great deal of hard work from a number of people. Our first debt - and a large one - is to the team of interviewers who carried out the main survey; Helen Bartram, Robin Hall, Ruth Simms, Lyn Snowden, Rosemary Watson, Leila Woolf and Angela Zvesper. They gave a commitment and attention to detail which cannot be explained by the relatively modest financial incentives which we were able to offer.

Eileen Sutcliffe, Tony Weekes and Geoff Hardman did a great deal for us in processing the data. Tony Weekes is mainly responsible for Appendix 1. Norman Ellis, John Henderson, John Horder, Donald Irvine, Brian Jarman and Gavin Mooney made helpful comments on proposals and drafts, and the contribution of Donald Fairclough was enormous at a critical point. Lise Rochaix helped with the drafting of the questionnaire for the pilot study, and we are grateful to Amanda Gott for drawing the figures.

Our colleagues Alan Maynard, Alan Williams and Ken Wright made useful comments; we would particularly wish to acknowledge our debt to Roy Carr-Hill in clarifying our thinking. Thanks are also due to Elaine Porter for help with many financial details and to Sal Cuthbert, Kerry Atkinson, Sally Baker, Sue White and Vanessa Windass for their constant good humour in the face of unreasonable typing requests.

We would like to thank the Economic and Social Research Council and the Health Promotion Research Trust for their financial support. The staff of the HPRT have been most helpful. Bob King gave us assistance at the beginning and Chris Henshall has given us unstinting support. Clare Freeman was most helpful in preparing the text for publication.

A final thank you must go to the many family doctors who gave their time so freely; and to Anne and Henry for their constant support and encouragement throughout the study.

York, August 1988

1 Introduction

In Britain, general practitioners are independent contractors within the National Health Service. Since the Family Doctor Charter (British Medical Association, 1965), general practice has become an increasingly popular choice for medical students, and has embodied an ideal which has attracted many of the most able and committed medical graduates over the past twenty years.

Yet until recently much writing about primary care was prescriptive and optimistic, describing best practice and advocating the extension of primary care as an obvious way of providing a more accessible and a more cost effective service to the public (British Medical Association, 1984). Government policy statements paid tribute to the successes of primary care in Britain and promised an expansion (Department of Health and Social Security, 1986).

The quality of service provision by general practitioners had received little attention until the publication of documents by the Royal College of General Practitioners (Royal College of General Practitioners, 1985 and 1985a) and the British Medical Association (British Medical Association, 1984). These documents advocated examination of the way in which general practice is organised, to increase "quality" of care to patients. They anticipated the government White Paper (Department of Health and Social Security, 1987), which gave particular emphasis to making the general practitioner service accountable to patients and suggested ways of improving services.

The results achieved in practice have seemed in many ways to fall far short of the ideals. There may be much commitment by individuals but the primary care system in Britain exhibits some signs of malaise.

The level of resources used both in the family doctor service and more widely in primary care has risen sharply compared to the hospital services. From 1978/9 to 1985/6 spending on the general medical services rose by 57.1 per cent in volume terms; spending on primary care as a whole rose by 27.8 per cent and on hospital and community health services by 4.5 per cent (Table 1.1).

Table 1.1
Expenditure on the primary care margins (England)
(£ million 1985/86 prices)

	1978-9	1985-6	% change
General Medical Services	711	1117	57.1
Pharmaceutical Services	1258	1549	23.1
Acute out-patients	930.5	1058.6	13.8
Health visiting	120.5	148.9	23.6
District nursing	223.1	292.6	31.1
School health services	136.5	155.3	13.8
Community midwifery	59.3	73.0	23.1
Total FPS-HCHS* primary care	3438.9	4394.4	27.8
Other HCHS	7722.4	7881.0	2.0
Total HCHS	9192.3	9609.4	4.5

* Family Practitioner Services-Hospital and Community Health Services.
Source : House of Commons Social Services Committee (1987); Office of Health Economics, 1987.

Over the period of the Family Doctor Charter the number of new out-patient attendances per 1000 population rose from 311 in 1966 to 404 in 1985. The long wait for a sequel to the Green Paper on primary care reflected the policy deadlock on a number of key issues: on the payment system of family doctors; on their future relationships with the nursing profession; and on the future role of primary care relative to other services (Department of Health and Social Security, 1986). The focus of government policy for several years has been on the hospital and community health services and the new philosophy of general management has stopped short of general practice. Now with the new White Paper there are signs of change - but there are many difficulties in the way of making more effective use of resources (Bosanquet, 1986).

There has been very little evaluation of the benefits of increased spending on a number of closely related programmes such as general medical services, out-patient services and community nursing. The expansion took place at a time when there were many criticisms of the effectiveness of these services, for example, of "unnecessary" out-patient appointments. (Marsh, 1982). Given the importance of budgetary constraints in the National Health Service there has been surprisingly little attention to these issues of resource use on the primary care margins.

General practitioners essentially operate as small businesses, providing services to all the patients on their lists. Large partnerships have a considerable financial turnover. Income for the partners is derived from the practice 'profits'. General practitioners have some advantages over most owners of small businesses in that they are unlikely to become unemployed and are members of the National Health Service superannuation scheme. They are in an ambivalent position as independent contractors working for a monopoly. Their decisions are also affected by the web of rules set by the Family Practitioner Committees (FPCs) of which there are 90 in England.

The current situation

The Family Practitioner Committees are responsible for financing the primary care services in their areas. Total expenditure on the family doctor service is part of a larger flow of payments administered by Family Practitioner Committees. They also cover general dental, general ophthalmic and pharmaceutical services. The proportions of spending accounted for by these services together with the changes in shares since 1965 are shown in Table 1.2.

Table 1.2
National Health Service gross expenditure and Family Practitioner Service expenditure : percentage composition of totals

	1965	1987
Hospital services	60.4	58.0
Community Health	10.3	6.4
General Medical	7.8	7.5
General Dental	5.1	4.3
General Ophthalmic	1.6	0.7
Pharmaceutical	11.1	10.3
Other	3.7	12.8

Source: Office of Health Economics, 1987.

The amounts spent on the general medical services have not been large enough to bring into play the full battery of controls which has developed on public expenditure since 1976. But they have not been small enough to be ignored. The intermittent attentions accorded to Family Practitioner Service expenditure within the budgetary system may well have done less than justice to the role of general practitioners in generating spending indirectly through referral and prescribing. These well used measures of general practitioners' own expenditure of the type set out in Table 1.2 do not really deal adequately with the wider impact of general practitioners' decisions.

Table 1.3
Numbers of unrestricted general practitioners and average list sizes

Year	Number (England & Wales)	Average list size (England)
1951	17,135	2,554
1955	18,832	2,283
1960	19,905	2,287
1965	20,014	2,412
1970	20,357	2,460
1975	21,667	2,365
1980	23,184	2,247
1985	25,558	2,059
1986*	25,901	2,032

*estimated
Source: Office of Health Economics, 1987.

Table 1.4
Percentage distribution of unrestricted principals by size of practice, UK

Size of practice	1951	1970	1982	1986
Single handed	43	21	13	11
2 partners	33	25	17	16
3 partners	15	26	23	21
4 partners	6	16	20	19
5 partners	2	7	14	15
6+ partners	1	5	14	17

Source: Office of Health Economics, 1987.

The numbers of general practitioners have been increasing, as shown in Table 1.3. This increase in general practitioner numbers has been accompanied by a gradual fall in average list size. At the same time, partnership size has been increasing (Table 1.4) encouraged by the payment of the Group Practice Allowance for practices of three or more partners as part of the Family Doctor Charter (British Medical Association, 1965). The overall trend has therefore been towards larger practices with smaller list sizes.

At the same time, the age distribution of general practitioners has been changing (Table 1.5). The numbers of female general practitioners have been increasing (Table 1.6). Although only 7 per cent of the United Kingdom population were born abroad (1983 figures), 23 per cent of general practitioners were born overseas (Table 1.7).

Table 1.5
Percentage of General Practitioners by age group, England

Age (years)	1965	1975	1985
less than 30	5	7	8
30-39	26	24	32
40-49	31	29	25
50-59	23	26	22
60-69	13	11	10
70 +	2	3	2

Source: Department of Health and Social Security, 1987a.

Table 1.6
Percentage distribution of general practitioners by sex, England

Year	Male	Female
1968	90	10
1975	86	14
1985	79	21
[2001*	72	28]

*projected

Source: Department of Health and Social Security, 1987a.

Table 1.7
Percentage distribution of general practitioners by place of birth

	1968	1983
Great Britain	77	73
Ireland	10	4
Elsewhere	13	23

Source: Fry, 1986.

This, then, is the background against which this study of general practice is set. But what patterns of decision making by individual practices lie behind these broad aggregates? The question gains in importance as the stock of general practitioners has become more varied and younger.

The development of general practice in Britain has usually been seen in terms of aggregate changes in practice structure, list size, shares of expenditure and the background characteristics of general practitioners. These figures are usually presented in terms of slow trends over decades during which list sizes fall, the incidence of larger practices increases, and the share of general medical services falls as a proportion of National Health Service spending. These changes have been recorded above. This study aims to go beyond this type of description and to look at the decisions made by individual practices which lie behind these aggregate changes. In pursuit of this aim, the study will stress the variations which persist rather than just the uniformity of the aggregate movements. Thus, although it is true that there are more larger practices, later evidence will show that the degree of change has been very uneven. There are many areas - especially older industrial areas where the need for medical and preventive services is greatest - where there has not been a major change to larger practices. The survey presents new evidence on how the aggregate movements are affected by many different decisions on practice strategy and on the forces shaping those decisions.

The model of general practice

This study is an attempt to determine how economic considerations influence practice decisions at the local level. There are proposals being made for possible extensions of the general practitioner's role, especially in the area of prevention (Department of Health and Social Security, 1987). In this White Paper there are important proposals for the revision of the Family Doctor Charter, for example the introduction of additional fee for service items. Yet there is little evidence on how general practitioners actually take decisions which will help in assessing the impact of these proposals.

The benefits of improvement to some minimum standard have often been treated as self evident. As an editorial in the Lancet put it:

> "No randomised trial is necessary to show that GPs working from their own front parlours or squalid lockup shops, in isolation, without office or nursing staff, and treating all the costs of a public service from their own pockets, make less effective use of their long and costly training than GPs working in groups, assisted by secretaries and nurses, in purpose built premises, with most of the costs met directly by the state". (Lancet, 1984)

What factors motivate general practitioners to improve their premises, to employ more staff and provide more services? If contributory factors could be ascertained, then the way is open for encouragement of all general practitioners to improve their services to patients, for, as Butler and Calnan put it:

> "GPs are not passive responders to circumstance, they are active creators of their working environment. They can usually choose the types of premises in which they will work, the size and composition of their practice teams, the emphasis they will give to training, research or prevention, the extent of their commitments outside their practices, the amount of equipment they will buy, the length of their booking intervals, the readiness with which they will undertake home visits the forms of record-keeping they will adopt, the arrangements they will make for out-of-hours cover, and a multitude of other facets of the day-to-day work of their practices". (Butler and Calnan, 1987)

Much has been written about changes in health policy and incentives at the national level: this study looks at the local response.

Figure 1.1 summarises the model of general practice which has been used to test hypotheses in this study.

The general practitioner characteristics are mainly personal factors such as age, sex, nationality, but also include other variables such as membership of professional organisations (British Medical Association, Royal College of General Practitioners), take-up of outside posts, as well as the time spent in the existing practice and whether the doctor is working in a full-time or part-time capacity. Data are available from the survey on all these variables. These personal characteristics would be expected to have a strong influence on decisions made within the practice. The payment system will also affect practice decisions on services, staffing and premises. The decision to become a training practice may well be influenced by the educational achievements of the practice partners, or by the way in which practice finances are organised. The capitation fee element in the payment system influences list size, and there are proposals in the White Paper (Department of Health and Social Security, 1987) to bring about a rise in the capitation fee element from the current 47 per cent of net income to 50 per cent.

The last set of factors affecting practice decisions is to do with the location of the practice. The survey has selected seven areas of England with differing demographic and social characteristics. The problems and decisions faced by practices will vary with the local environment. For example, a practice in a deprived inner city area may well not have an appointment system because most patients do not have access to telephones, whereas in more affluent areas, an appointment system has become accepted as the norm. Doctors have to adapt the organisation of their

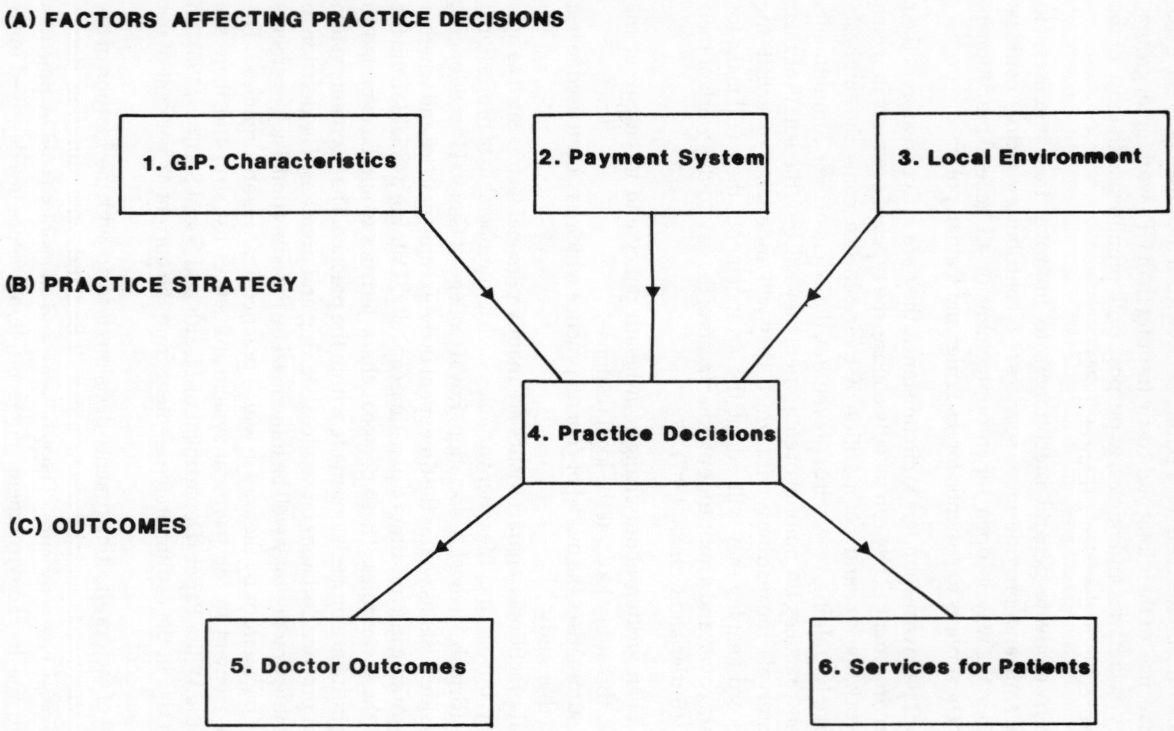

Figure 1.1 The model of general practice

practices to local conditions. In rural areas practices have to organise their own out-of-hours cover, whereas those in urban areas have the choice of a deputising service should they wish to make use of it.

It is debatable how far the environment influences the general practitioner or vice versa. It is clear that some general practitioners relish the challenge of working in an inner city environment and actually choose to work there, but in other cases doctors find themselves in this type of area because positions in other more environmentally pleasant areas are harder to come by. The study provides some evidence on the types of practices located in different types of areas.

'GP characteristics', the payment system and the local environment trigger decisions on practice structure. The study is mainly concerned with causation, the impact of the variables in the first three boxes in Figure 1.1 on practice decisions. Practices have to make decisions on partnership size, staffing, use of branch surgeries, dispensing, off-duty cover, record systems, equipment, and whether to become a training practice. Data have been collected on all of these variables.

Which of these practice decisions on strategy have the greatest financial impact and are measurable? The study has looked in detail at the financing of practice premises, particularly the cost rent scheme (described in Chapter two) which allows practices to improve their premises. In spite of the reimbursements under the cost rent scheme, general practitioners still incur costs. The cost rent scheme does, however, allow doctors to provide a favourable working environment for their patients as well as for themselves, and they gain an appreciating asset in the form of owned premises. The decision, therefore, to take part in a cost rent scheme has important consequences financially and is directly affected by factors such as the age of the partners, practice location and a desire for improvement. Similarly, the employment of a practice nurse has been taken, in this study, as an indicator of the desire to provide a better service to patients, but one which again involves costs to the practice.

Thirdly, participation in the training scheme means that a practice has to reach and maintain certain standards and be subject to external audit. The decision to be a training practice therefore implies that a practice has reached certain standards. There is some financial recompense for having a trainee, but there are also opportunity costs for the time taken to train the trainee.

This study therefore pays close attention to these three factors of general practice strategy; use of the cost rent scheme; employment of a practice nurse; participation in the training scheme, to define a group of practices, designated "innovators", having two or more of the above characteristics, which most closely approximate the approved model of general practice. Practices which have none of the three characteristics have been designated "traditionalists" and the remaining practices "intermediates". Traditionalists may be practising first class medicine but they are doing it without team support or external audit and in older premises. These decisions on practice strategy lead to outcomes for the general practitioners in terms of net and gross incomes and capital costs. They also have to face up to outcomes in terms of workload and all these outcomes shape their views of the future.

Practice strategy has implications for patients too. The study has not collected patient views, nor has it collected information on consultation rates or referral rates. It has, however, collected data on factors which affect patients directly, such as provision of special clinics, family planning services, obstetric services and home confinements. Data have also been collected on the use of age/sex registers and appointment systems, which although not directly perceived by patients, do have implications for their satisfaction with the services provided. Outcomes for patients in terms of the quality of advice and satisfaction have not been collected.

The main variables covered in the six boxes of Figure 1.1 are summarised in Table 1.8.

Practice strategy is defined in terms of interrelated decisions on premises, size of partnership, staffing and equipment. In looking at practice decisions the study concentrates on the following hypotheses.

(1) Practice strategy will be influenced by the personal characteristics, professional contact and motivation of the family doctor. Professional motivation cannot be measured directly but decisions made by partners about membership of professional organisations or participation in the Vocational Training Scheme will provide some indirect evidence.

(2) Practice strategy will be influenced by the local environment of the practice. This will have an impact both through demography and through changes in social composition. Areas of rising population will be expected to have an increasing list size generating an increasing income to practices. In more middle class areas there may be more patient pressure to improve premises and to provide new services.

(3) Practice strategy will affect the financial pressures facing a practice. Those practices which have been most active in changing their structure and in developing services will face the greatest financial pressures.

The hypotheses imply that a mix of professional and economic incentives will affect a practice. Personal characteristics might sometimes reflect different professional incentives. Thus membership of professional organisations may give some clue to family doctors' views of their own role. The age of doctors gives some clue to the generation they come from and the kind of professional experiences they have been through. Ethnic background may well reflect different experiences in training and views of how the job might be done. Personal characteristics may also affect economic interest especially in the case of age, where younger doctors may have a stronger incentive to invest, but the influence of personal characteristics is likely to reflect predominantly those of professional incentives. The qualifications, the associations and the attitudes to co-operation with others, bring mainly intangible returns and add more to cost and responsibility than to direct financial reward.

The main effect of economic incentives may well be through the local environment. The local environment promises returns in terms of income, and local comparisons within a general practice 'market' will encourage initiation of new strategies. But the impact of the local environment will also be affected by differences of intrinsic motivation as well as by age. Thus in some unpromising areas some groups of partners will show a very strong motivation to raise income and to develop practices. The local environment may also affect the professional atmosphere and professional standards within a peer group of local doctors.

Table 1.8

The model of general practice

(A) Factors affecting practice decisions

1. General Practitioner characteristics

Age, Sex
Ethnic background
Length of service
Nature of contract (full or part-time)
Membership of professional organisations
Outside posts

2. Payment system

Level of income
Structure of income: Incentives through fees for service
Staff reimbursement

3. Practice location and local environment

Social characteristics of the Family Practitioner Committee area
Social characteristics of the practice catchment area
Changes in the local population

(B) Practice strategy

4. Practice decisions

List size
Partnership size
Staffing (including nurses)
Equipment
Obligations as a dispensing practice
Participation in Vocational Training Scheme
Premises (including cost rent scheme)
Off-duty cover
Type of contract
Record systems

(C) Outcomes

5. Outcomes for Doctors

Gross and net incomes
Expense ratios
Capital costs
Workload and pressure of work

6. Services for patients

Appointment systems
Age/sex registers
Special clinics
Type of family planning service
Maternity services

There is a common belief that the incentives facing the family doctor are mainly perverse - those who develop their practices will find little net return. The third hypothesis is set up in order to test this common assumption: are the rewards to innovation consistently low or negative or can local environment operate to create larger rewards in some areas? The survey evidence gives the opportunity of testing out the possibilities.

There now follows a more detailed discussion of the variables used in the model.

The background to the study

Factors affecting practice decisions

1. *General practitioner characteristics* These characteristics would be expected to have a large influence on doctors' decisions. Age and length of service are closely related variables but ones which require separate investigation. Female doctors form an increasing proportion of the total and could be expected to have distinctive ideas about practice organisation. Family doctors might choose to join various professional organisations and their decision might give some pointer to their professional attitudes, as was found in an earlier study by Cartwright and Anderson (Cartwright and Anderson, 1981) where membership of the Royal College of General Practitioners was significantly related to differences in decisions. The type of contract used could also influence decisions. The use of part-time contracts is increasingly common in service industries and the effects of part-time status on practice style need investigating.

2. *The payment system* A practice can make several decisions based on the payment system (described in detail in Chapter Two) aimed at maximising income. A practice could aim to increase list size and so achieve a higher capitation income; it could aim to increase fee for service income by providing more services to patients, possibly in the form of clinics; or it could reduce costs.

EFFECT OF INCREASED FEE FOR SERVICE INCOME Practices which aim to increase income face certain problems in that fee for service relates to certain patient groups only, mainly families with young children. If these are few in the practice area then opportunities will be reduced. If a practice has a low coverage of these eligible patients, it may be able to increase coverage and raise income for a year or two, but after that, progress will be slowed. Some practices in some areas do receive information on client group coverage and levels of fee for service income, but this is patchy and not all practices keep their own records. The ability to increase income from fee for service is therefore a practice decision, the effects of which are dependent on the location of the practice.

EFFECT OF REDUCING COSTS Costs can be reduced in two ways. A small traditional practice could operate in older premises, and save on indirectly reimbursed costs such as heating and cleaning. It could also avoid staffing costs and in effect operate in obsolete premises providing its patients with amenities below generally acceptable levels. Practices which have invested in new premises could achieve cost containment by efficient management. Since the payment system is based on average costs incurred by all general practitioners, any practice which had costs below the average would add significantly to net income, since practice costs range from 20 to 40 per cent of gross income. A practice which reduced costs from 35 per cent to 25 per cent of gross income could add approximately £4,000 per partner to net annual income. This is equivalent to an additional 700 patients per list. However, such cost containment would be much more difficult for practices which had invested in new premises.

3. *The local environment* Within the National Health Service it is difficult for a practice to shift location except within a Family Practitioner Committee area and even then such moves are rare. Many practices stay at the same location for decades. The size of partnership may change gradually but once a partner has moved in, he or she is almost irremovable. Decisions on buildings and branch premises affect the outputs that can be produced by the practice in terms of the number of partners and the services offered.

Such decisions will affect the demand for the practice's services as well as its income and costs. If a practice is located in an area of expanding population this will lead to more demand from families with children. Thus, practice income will be raised through fees for service and the effects of rising list size as the local population expands. The size and nature of the practice premises will affect its costs and the net income of the partners. Thus, investment strategy affects professional goals (by making it easier or more difficult to provide services) and the financial return to the doctor. This return will be affected by the local environment through changes in local population and by the extent of local competition as represented by the ease of entry of new practices. Practice location will also affect initial recruitment to practices, with greater pressure on vacancies in the more affluent and attractive areas.

Practice strategy

1. *List and partnership size* What incentives do practices face which might affect decisions on strategy? Incentives to high list size are weak. Table 1.9 shows how income increases with increasing list size. There will also be increasing costs in terms of time and effort involved in increasing list size which should be offset against the apparent income gains, and in any case, marginal income falls sharply as list size increases, from £25.20 per patient for the first 1000 to £9.50 for additional patients.

Partnerships have increased in size. How far does this reflect economic incentives as well as official encouragement? There is evidence from Canada that group practices had higher profit margins (Boan, 1966). To what extent are larger practices in Britain likely to be more 'profitable'? Doctors in group practices of three or more partners get paid a special allowance, currently £1,355 a year: but more important are the cost-sharing and risk-sharing effects of larger practices. A doctor in single handed practice who employs two staff, a nurse (part-time) and a receptionist, would incur gross costs of £10,000. After the Family Practitioner Committee contribution of £7,000 and a tax allowance of £1,500, the net cost to him or her would be £1,500, all of which would fall on the doctor's income. A five partner practice would have to employ ten staff before the same effect on the net income of each partner, and on average such a practice would employ only five staff. There is also a risk-sharing effect in that investment in new premises would be spread over a number of partners in larger practices. Against this would have to be set greater difficulties in management, coordination and patient access in large practices. In one area, two practices of six partners decided recently to break into separate partnerships as a result of difficulties of this kind (Siddy, 1987). Thus it is not possible at present to say what is the most economic scale of practice. It is clear that doctors in single handed practices have lower incomes and work longer hours - 41 hours per week as against 38 for doctors in partnerships (Department of Health and Social Security, 1987b). There may well be gains in cost-sharing and risk-sharing between two and five partners but at some size of practice the problems of coordination, adequacy of premises and patient access may lead to diseconomies of scale.

2. *Staffing* Practices are also making medium term decisions on staffing. In 1984 there were 30,000 staff employed by practices, a ratio of 1.062 employees per doctor (Department of Health and Social Security, 1987). These commitments are often described in terms of 'teamwork'. One effect will be on the doctor's own working hours (Department of Health and Social Security, 1987b). This may in part be because of additional work in supervision and management, but the doctors may also be doing more themselves. The proportion of doctors who had a nurse working in the practice either on an employed or an attached basis rose from 12 per cent in 1964 to 84 per cent in 1977. Some doctors were undertaking a wider range of tasks, especially where the nurses were employed (Cartwright, 1967; Cartwright and Anderson, 1981). Doctors were more likely to undertake procedures such as fitting intrauterine devices, excising cysts, taking blood or stitching cuts if there was a nurse in the practice. Attachment of other professionals also seemed to change the pattern of activity. Local case studies have suggested that such attachments lead to increased referral to these workers and to changes in attitude (Horder, Bosanquet and Stocking, 1986). Nine doctors in a South London group practice with a four year history of social work attachments were asked how the attachments had affected their work. All considered the attachments to have been very helpful and agreed that the social workers had increased their awareness of the patients' psychosocial problems (Williams and Clare, 1979). An evaluation of a one year attachment of three community psychiatric nurses to three group practices in Oxford found a redistribution of the doctors' workloads. The 'level of involvement' of each doctor with patients was scored before and after the referral and found to drop by 50 per cent (Harker, Leopoldt and Robinson, 1976). A study by Lyall, of nine practices in North West London working with a marriage guidance counsellor, found consultations reduced by a third, prescriptions by nearly a half and prescribing of psychotropic drugs by a third (Lyall, 1979). The employment or attachment of staff to a practice 'team' does not therefore simply lead to the delegation of tasks: it leads to changes in workload and in the range of tasks that are undertaken. The most important effects are on the doctor's own role.

3. *Equipment* Levels of capitalisation of general practice in terms of equipment and information technology have been low, but these resources are likely to become more important as the service mix and technology change. Normally, technology and working capital are important ways of increasing efficiency in service industries

Table 1.9
Variations in basic general practitioner income by list sizes
(from April 1st 1987)

	1000 patients	2000 patients	2500 patients	3000 patients
Basic practice allowance (flat rate)	7,850	7,850	7,850	7,850
100-999 patients at £6.97 each	6,273	6,273	6,273	6,273
Capitation fees :				
Under 65 at £7.55	6,478	12,956	16,202	19,434
*65-75 at £9.80	911	1,823	2,274	2,734
75+ at £12.05	590	1,180	1,470	1,771
Supplementary practice allowance	1,575	1,575	1,575	1,575
First 100 patients	315	315	315	315
100-999 at £1.40 each	1,260	1,260	1,260	1,260
Fee for each patient over 1000 at £1.54	-	1,540	2,310	3,080
	25,252	34,772	39,529	44,292
Average income per patient	25.2	17.4	15.8	14.8
Marginal income per patient	25.2	9.5	9.5	9.5

* assuming a normal age ratio of 9.3 per cent aged 65-74 and 4.9 per cent aged over 75

Source: Department of Health and Social Security (1987) and authors' calculations.

and these have become even more significant through changes which have made technology much more accessible to small enterprises. Twenty years ago the use of computing and information processing was limited to government and to other large organisations such as banks. Now small firms as well as households have access to powerful and inexpensive means of information processing. Family doctors are only now beginning to share in the benefit of this change and the scope for computer use in general practice is large.

4. *Dispensing* As well as decisions made by practices about their own resources in terms of time, capital and staffing, general practitioners are also committing other resources through their decisions on referral to hospital and in prescribing. These aspects of general practice are outside the scope of this study, but dispensing

practices located in rural areas, are able to make substantial profits from this activity. There are few dispensing practices in urban areas.

5. *Training* Since 1981, all applicants for practice vacancies must have experienced at least one year's vocational training, as well as two year's hospital experience. In 1986 there were 2,000 trainees representing 80 per cent of all general practitioners. In addition, 10 per cent of established general practitioners were trainers. The decision to become a training practice is one affecting all the partners although only one partner may be a trainer. Sufficient space and time have to be allocated to training and certain standards have to be met, but there is a financial incentive and the bonus of an additional member of the practice team.

6. *Premises* The decision to invest in new practice premises is a major one and has far-reaching implications for the practice, not the least of which is financial. Although finance is readily available for premises under the cost rent and other schemes (see Chapter Two), with what are effectively interest free loans, capital still has to be repaid. This may cause disincentives to leave a practice, cause difficulty in entering a practice and be a problem for part-time partners. However, most general practitioners under the age of fifty years now practice from premises which have been built or improvedover the past twenty years.

7. *Off-duty cover* Practices can either decide to provide this cover themselves or to employ a deputising service. Their decisions may be a clue as to whether practices wish to minimise direct financial costs, but in many, particularly rural areas, deputising services are simply not available.

Outcomes

1. *General practitioner outcomes* These include incomes and costs, but also workload and job satisfaction. In the past, general practitioner workload was almost entirely set by demand. There were certain surgery hours and intervals between consultations. There was also a demand for home visits. The content of the consultation was traditional with the emphasis on the relief of symptoms, or on diagnosis. For a number of reasons family doctors now have much greater discretion over the content of consultations and over the pattern of services. One reason is that there is more time available in which to make changes. Working hours have fallen. Actual working hours averaged 38 per week in 1985 which is rather less than the average for full-time employed male adults and much less than the average for the self-employed (Department of Employment, 1986). In addition, there are hours on call, but these again are reduced compared with the past by the use of deputising services, and probably by a reduced number of night calls because of improved methods for the treatment of asthma and bronchitis. Within surgery hours, the number of consultations which each doctor has to face each working week has fallen: the average length of consultation has risen from six to 8.24 minutes (Department of Health and Social Security, 1987b). Thus the family doctor has more time to use on a discretionary basis and more ways in which this time could be used, ranging from greater leisure to different kinds of treatment and preventive programmes.

The amount of discretionary time available to each general practitioner will vary with individual choice and with list size. Working hours are slightly longer and consultations shorter as list size increases (Department of Health and Social Security, 1987b) but the most significant difference is in pressure of demand between regions - the regional range in consultation rates varied between 3.7 in Oxford to 5.1 in Wales. A general practitioner in Oxford with a list size of 2,100 will have 7,800 consultations per year while a general practitioner in Wales will have 10,700 (Office of Health Economics, 1987). There will be local variations in the amount of discretionary time available as well as individual variations due to the general practitioner's own preference.

2. *Patient outcomes* Patient outcomes in this study include services provided by the practice, including clinics or preventive programmes. Practices have some discretion on their style and range of care. Some of the clinics are traditional, specialising in ante-natal care or immunisation, but there are now many other possibilities. There could be special help to client groups, such as developmental paediatrics as suggested in the White Paper (Department of Health and Social Security, 1987), or for people with particular kinds of illness such as hypertension or diabetes. These special areas of activity usually involve an element of prevention or anticipatory care. They involve practice organisation to identify and contact certain age groups and diagnostic conditions. These activities also involve teamwork so that they are very different in their implications for the practice than the older, demand-led services.

Earlier studies of general practice

Earlier studies have tended to concentrate on specific aspects of general practice. Butler (1980) and more recently, Butler & Calnan (1987) looked in detail at list sizes in general practice. This followed an earlier study on the geographical distribution of general practitioners (Butler, Bevan and Taylor, 1973). Metcalfe, Wilkin, Hodgkin, Hallam and Cooke (1983) looked at general practitioner case mix, comparing the inner city with more affluent areas in the process of care provided by a sample of general practitioners. Dowie's (1983) study of general practitioners and consultants was concerned with referral patterns, and Bowling (1981) looked at delegation in general practice. There have also been studies on teamwork in general practice (Marsh and Kaim-Caudle, 1976; Reedy *et al*, 1983) and numerous localised studies (Mair and Mair, 1959; Steen, 1967; Marsh and McNay, 1974; Pike, Beaumont and Clewett, 1981; Wilkin, Hallam, Leavey and Metcalfe, 1987). The Royal College of General Practitioners has also produced a number of relevant publications (Royal College of General Practitioner occasional papers numbers 12, 13, 15, 16, 19, 20 and 21).

The Collings Report (Collings, 1950) provided an overview of general practice at that time, and Cartwright and Marshall (1965) looked in detail at the work of a national sample of general practitioners, as did Irvine and Jeffreys in 1971 (Irvine and Jeffreys, 1971). Most recently there has been the study commissioned in response to a request by the Doctors' and Dentists' Review Body for better information about workload (Department of Health and Social Security, 1987b). However, the studies of Cartwright (1967) and of Cartwright and Anderson (1981) are particularly relevant to the present study.

These surveys provide a detailed picture of change in practices' methods of working over a period of thirteen years. In 1964 Cartwright interviewed 1,397 patients in twelve areas and sent a postal questionnaire to their general practitioners and the 1977 survey was on similar lines. These surveys provide a good picture of general practice during the first half of the Family Doctor Charter. The general conclusions were that practice structure had changed a good deal but with little change in attitudes and the range of work done. The Family Doctor Charter had given general practice greater stability and led to the employment of more staff, but the services provided, and the doctor-patient relationships, remained rather similar. There had been "major changes in the organisation of the general practitioner service alongside small and mainly insignificant changes in the basic relationship between patients and doctors" (Cartwright and Anderson, 1981). This study, like the earlier ones, could not look directly at the relationships between doctors and patients, but did provide some evidence of change in professional orientation over the last ten years. Changes in practice strategy have been considerable over the period and supply some evidence for greater response to incentives than was present in the earlier periods.

The economics of general practice - or even that of primary care - have received rather little attention from health economists. There has been some work on the demand for health care and much more on the immediate policy and budgetary problems of health systems. The supply side as a whole has had a smaller share of attention and most of this has gone to the problems of supply and cost of hospitals. The most widely read text book of health economics in the United Kingdom devotes two pages to the economics of primary care (Cullis and West, 1979). The main role of the general practitioner is seen in terms of screening or in decisions on referral. The behaviour of primary suppliers will depend on their objectives, on the payment system and on patient demand. A fee for service system will produce different levels of activity and different patterns of location from capitation payments. A fee for service system will encourage concentration in high income areas. Cullis and West conclude that:

> "clearly a more detailed model of general practice would be required to examine this issue further. However, to the extent that general practice is becoming more complex, e.g. through the introduction of nurses and diagnostic equipment, models of hospital behaviour may be relevant for the general practitioner." (Cullis and West, 1979).

The development of a distinctive economics of general practice has hardly been a priority in spite of the importance of the decisions taken by general practitioners in affecting the use of resources throughout the health care system.

The independent contractual status of the general practitioner used to be seen as an anomaly which reflected past political power rather than current function. However, increasing discussion of the possible role of internal markets in the National Health Service may make it a model of mixed enterprise for the future, rather than a survival from the past (Enthoven, 1985). Family doctors have had to make their own decisions on many issues and their response to incentives may help to show how internal markets might work in the National Health Service.

Models of medical behaviour

There has been one area of work which forms an exception to the general neglect: this is the work done in the United States on models of medical behaviour. How relevant is this work to the particular problems of general practice in Britain? Early work was carried out in the late 1960s and the early 1970s. The focus was on the rising price of physicians' services, and studies concentrated on the decisions about productivity made by physicians, and their response to rising demand for their services. The work of Feldstein showed that the pricing and use of physicians' services could best be understood by assuming that permanent excess demand prevailed:

> "sheltered by this excess demand, physicians have discretion over power to vary both their prices and the quantity of services which they supply." (Feldstein, 1970.)

Reinhardt concluded that physicians were inefficient in the sense that they did not employ the number of aides which would have allowed them to maximise their output (Reinhardt, 1972). He concluded that the average American physician could profitably employ about twice the number of aides currently employed and by doing so would have increased the hourly rate of output by about 25 per cent. Such an increase would add more to output than would be contributed by several years classes of young doctors graduating from medical school.

These conclusions were reached through analysis of the 'production function' - the relationships between the 'inputs' of and labour used by the doctors and their 'outputs' in terms of numbers of consultations. Thus Reinhardt's 'productivity' is measured in terms of the rate at which patients visit the doctor or the number of billings which could be made per year. The production function is then used to estimate changes in output with different levels and different combinations of inputs.

More recently, there have been attempts to introduce into the account a more realistic view of what physicians are producing. Doctors are not just interested in maximising income or turnover; they are acting as agents for the patient, with a professional obligation to try to organise the most appropriate care. The doctor's utility is affected not just by his own income but by whether he thinks he has carried out his role as agent for the patient. Pauly has concluded from a model which incorporates these agency effects that there is in fact, no necessary conflict between the agency relationship and the doctor's self interest (Pauly, 1980). The agency relationship may also help to explain why doctors do not do some of the things that economists think they ought to do, such as to employ aides. There may be a loss of relationship to the patient involved, in employing an aide, which outweighs any possible gain in monetary terms. However, much of the work done so far has been abstract. For example, Woodward and Warren Boulton looked at relative effects of financial incentives and professional ethics on appropriate care (Woodward and Warren Boulton, 1984). They accepted that physicians are affected by professional goals such as the desire to cure the sick and to achieve professional excellence as well as by financial incentives - but their view of how the balance is arrived at in practice remains vague.

The lesson of production function analysis would seem to be that much more attention needs to be paid to motivation - or variables such as "appropriate care" will remain abstractions. Production function analysis also has little to say about the effects of local environment on practices. Practices are deeply influenced by the area and setting in which they work. The survey aims to provide some evidence about area influences on decision-making.

Summary

Practices are under professional pressure to carry out a strategy which includes investment in new premises, participation in the vocational training scheme and use of additional staffing. Practices that carry out this strategy may not necessarily achieve high quality but they have shown a response to incentives and a willingness to make decisions.

The survey seeks to show how family doctors take decisions. It covers most of the practices in seven different areas of the country and looks at decisions from the doctor's point of view. Chapters 3 to 8 explain how this was done and give the detailed results. It is possible to test out predictions both about "innovation" and about "income". It can be predicted there will be more innovation in practices where the average age of the partners is lower, and also in larger practices where economic risks are spread over several partners. Innovation is likely to vary with the degree of professional contact. Income levels are likely to be higher in areas of expanding population. Less easy to predict are the relative effects of age and area variables. How far does the local area have an impact independent of the age distribution of the family doctors in the area? How far are there any substantial differences in income reflecting local practice strategy given the highly centralised character of the payment system?

2 The financial background

The family doctor is in an unusual situation. Government regulations and policies limit his or her options but within a broad framework, general practitioners now have considerable discretion in making decisions. This chapter examines the economic constitution within which family doctors now work and traces how this element of discretion has increased.

Historical background

There have been three main policy phases. From 1911 to 1948 there was the panel doctor system. From 1948 to 1965 there was the initial phase within the National Health Service, and from 1965 onwards there was the Family Doctor Charter. (British Medical Association, 1965). The watershed is usually seen as the introduction of the National Health Service, but this was far less of a change for the family doctor service than for the hospitals. There was a continuity both in the issues which came up under the panel system through the first stage of the National Health Service, and in the policy approach to them. The issues presented themselves in terms of changes in demand for services, in the supply of doctors, and in pay. The policy response involved changes in a simple payments system involving capitation fees, negotiated by national organisations. The panel doctor era saw rising demand, some rise in supply and a large increase in relative pay. Under the first phase of the National Health Service, demand increased, supply was static, and relative pay fell. The changes led to tension and conflict between government and the profession, expressed through national negotiations.

The Family Doctor Charter represented a transition to a very different phase in which there was a much greater range of policies and much more scope for initiative by practices. It was under the incentives set up by the Family Doctor Charter that practices became able to change their own patterns of service - rather than to be simply passive recipients of capitation fees.

1. *The panel system* Initially, the patient coverage of the panel doctor system was restricted to males aged between 16 and 70 employed in manual labour or in non-manual jobs with an income of less than £160 a year (Digby and Bosanquet, 1988). Various extensions, both in terms of income and of age raised coverage from 13.7m people in 1914 to 19.2 m in 1936. The effect of this was to increase both the supply of services and doctors' incomes. Numbers of insurance practitioners rose from 13,700 in 1920 to 19,060 by 1938. The most striking change under the panel system was in the average incomes of family doctors. The cost of living fell by some 7-10 per cent for a doctor's household between 1924 and 1936, so that in real terms, general practitioners were almost 50 per cent better off at the end of the inter-war period than at the beginning. What had been a profession with high rewards for a few but inadequate income for the majority was transformed in part by the panel system into one in which all qualified doctors could enjoy a reasonable income.

Some enterprising general practitioners saw that the key decision was whether to employ an assistant, since this permitted an increase in the maximum insurance list of the single-handed practitioner from 2,500 to 4,000 and allowed the doctor to reap economies of scale. The panel system provided some opportunities for entrepreneurship. However, there was little progress in improving premises, and much concern about the quality of care especially in the maternity services and in the treatment of patients with fractures (Honigsbaum, 1979). There were also changes in the demand for services. The panel system provided incentives for working class patients to consult the doctor much more frequently than hitherto. The level of basic activities was three times higher than had been expected. (Digby and Bosanquet, 1988)

2. *The National Health Service and the Welfare State 1948-65* The main controversies before the setting up of the National Health Service were about the future of the hospital service. The future of general practice was a relatively minor issue apart from the one question of the coverage of dependents. The National Health Service extended coverage to the whole population without changing the capitation method of payment in its fundamentals. There had been proposals to give general practitioners salaried status but these were not adopted, and they remained independent contractors. The majority were in single-handed or two partner practice. There was a slight amendment to the payment system by the introduction of a flat-rate practice allowance as well as the basic capitation payment.

The general effect of the National Health Service was to lower the status of general practitioners compared to what it had been under the national insurance system. Under the National Insurance Act of 1911 the general practitioner was the main figure. The hospital system was left to its own devices and specialist hospital treatment was readily available only in a few centres. The National Health Service was about the extension of specialist hospital treatment to all, and the main controversies were about the future employment and income of hospital consultants. Once the consultants had been persuaded to join the National Health Service the general practitioners had little choice but to follow. As well as extending coverage to the whole population, the National Health Service set up a payment system involving a pool out of which the general practitioners had to find their own costs as well as income. General practitioners also inherited premises, capital stock, and a structure of practices which reflected the stresses and expedients of the wartime period. In essence, the theme of reconstruction which affected levels of spending elsewhere in the social services and in industry passed the family doctor service by. The capitation system of payment did not give them any financial incentive to invest in new premises and the virtual disappearance of private practice removed the social incentive to improve premises which had been effective in a few areas.

The family doctor entered the National Health Service on unfavourable terms in relation to hospital doctors and the position worsened in the 1950s. The greater availability of specialist hospital treatment was the most obvious new benefit from the National Health Service. Hospital consultants were found for the first time outside the main metropolitan centres. Under the panel system the consultants had been dependent on general practitioners for referrals and income but now this was no longer so. Numbers of hospital doctors rose much more rapidly than those of general practitioners and it became difficult to recruit to general practice.

The relations between the Ministry and the profession in the 1950s were dominated by one issue and one issue alone - that of pay. At the beginning of the decade, the Danckwerts Award (Ross, 1952) gave family doctors a substantial increase, after the earlier Spens Report (Ministry of Health, 1946) had left many issues unresolved. But it took more than ten years to set up a Review Body to adjudicate on a regular basis. The Pilkington Commission (Cabinet Office, 1960) recommended that the pool system should be retained but that the level of payment should be increased. For the future it recommended the setting up of a Review Body to determine pay levels. The only uses of fees for services were to be for temporary residents and for maternity services, and the only encouragement to invest in premises was a small contribution to the pool for group practice loans.

At the beginning of the National Health Service it was implied that the development of health centres would be important for family doctors. There was to be an alliance between the independent contractor and public investment through health centres. The health centre was to supply the investment element for which there was no incentive in the payment system, but in practice, health centres did not materialise and the policy was a failure. Fear of local government control was a large part of the reason for this and by 1963 only 26 health centres had been built.

The drift in the 17 years from 1948 to 1965 brought about the worst crisis which the family doctor service had known since 1910-11. As well as discontent about pay, two reports in the 1960s; the Porritt Report, (Medical Services Review Committee, 1962) and the Gillie Report (Ministry of Health, 1968) had presented a much more favourable view of the outlook for general practice. The Reports affirmed clearly, that good general practice was essential to good medicine and to the future of the National Health Service. They recommended a reduction in list size and the development of primary care teams and took a more critical view of the payments system. The Gillie Report made complementary recommendations on the extension of vocational training and the development of university departments of General Practice. The thinking behind these reports seemed to have provided most of the substance for the Family Doctor Charter which was agreed in 1965, (British Medical Association, 1965) thus ending the seventeen years of drift.

3. *The Family Doctor Charter* The Family Doctor Charter, narrowly defined, had the following main characteristics.

(1) It separated income from expenses, so that there were much greater incentives to invest in premises and to incur costs to make practices more attractive to patients. It also changed the payments system so that the capitation payment was less important, and basic practice allowances unrelated to list size were more important. In effect the incentive to very long lists was reduced.

(2) It encouraged practices to employ various kinds of supporting staff such as receptionists, secretaries and practice nurses.

(3) There were specific encouragements to group practice and to larger practices.

(4) There was a new General Practice Finance Corporation set up to encourage investment in general practice premises.

(5) There were some experiments with fees for service. In 1965 these were confined to payments for immunisation - but were later extended to cover payments for cervical cytology and for family planning. Some payment for maternity work had been made since 1960.

(6) There were special payments for doctors in "designated areas" in order to bring about a more equal distribution of general practitioners. (Butler, Bevan and Taylor, 1973.)

(7) Financial incentives were introduced to encourage the development of vocational training.

The Charter is usually seen in terms of incentives to change in practice structure, but it was also linked to other policies such as those of increasing manpower, equalising list size and encouraging vocational training. It was not only that the payment system became more complex: in a whole range of ways, practices had to face up to choice.

The structure of income and costs

Under the Family Doctor Charter, family doctors received an "average net remuneration" decided in successive Review Body reports produced annually. The elements in a general practitioner's pay are made up of capitation fees reflecting the number and age of the patients on the doctor's list; allowances, such as basic practice and supplementary practice allowances meant to cover provision of basic medical services and out-of-hours- cover respectively; and item of service fees which are more directly under the control of the general practitioners and cover maternity services, family planning, vaccination and immunisation, and cervical cytology, among others. In addition, income may be increased by private fees e.g. cremation fees, life insurance examinations etc. and by hospital and other part-time appointments.

Practice expenses are reimbursed directly by the Family Practitioner Committee for items such as surgery rent and rates (100 per cent) and ancillary staff salaries (70 per cent). Other expenses are covered by the payments made by Family Practitioner Committees which are intended to cover average practice costs found in a national sample of practice accounts. Table 2.1 sets out expenditure on general practice by Family Practitioner Committees in 1983-84.

Table 2.1
Expenditure on allowances and fees by Family Practitioner Committees1983-84

	£m	Percentage of total
Allowances	275	31.1
Capitation fees	379	42.8
Night visit fees	11	1.2
Vaccination and immunisation fees	14	1.6
Cervical cytology fees	3	0.3
Family planning	24	2.7
Maternity	4	0.4
Dispensing payments	111	12.5
Allowances for Vocational Training Scheme	37	4.2
Other payments	27	3.0
Total	885	100.0

Source: Department of Health and Social Security, 1986.

The Review Body system originated after the findings of the Pilkington Commission (Cabinet Office, 1960). The aims of the Review Body on Doctors' and Dentists' Remuneration were: (1) to avoid disputes over pay between the government and the medical profession, (2) to give assurance to the medical profession that their living standards would not be depressed by arbitrary government action, (3) to ensure that tax payers did not pay more than they should towards the payment of doctors (and dentists).

The expenses element is determined from a yearly sample survey of doctors' practice accounts supplied by the Inland Revenue to a joint technical committee of the General Medical Services Committee (GMSC) of the British Medical Association, and the Department of Health and Social Security.

1. *Capitation fees* These constitute the major payment received by general practitioners. A basic fee is paid for each patient under the age of 65, a higher rate for patients aged 65-74, and the highest rate for patients over the age of 75. The payment received by each doctor or practice is clearly dependent on list size, which has been falling

slowly in recent years. (see Table 1.3). General practitioners practising in areas which attract large numbers of retired people will receive more income from capitation fees.

2. *Basic practice allowance* Most general practitioners receive this allowance which is paid in full to all those with at least 1000 patients on their list and who spend at least 20 hours per week on patient care. It is paid at a reduced rate to doctors with smaller list sizes. The allowance is intended to cover the basic running costs involved in the care of patients and is the largest allowance paid to general practitioners.

3. *Supplementary practice allowance* This allowance, paid to most general practitioners, is for providing out of hours cover.

4. *Other allowances* These include the designated area allowance paid to general practitioners working in under-doctored areas, and the group practice allowance paid to encourage doctors to work in groups and to reduce the number of singlehanded practices. Other allowances include the postgraduate training allowance and the training grant received by general practitioner trainers. The rural practice allowance is paid to general practitioners practising in rural areas as a contribution towards their greater travelling costs. There are also seniority allowances.

5. *Item of service fees* These are paid for specific services, the doctor completing a claim form and submitting it to the Family Practitioner Committee. The fee can be claimed for each injection when a child is vaccinated against diphtheria, tetanus, whooping cough, measles, rubella, or given oral polio vaccine. The fee for performing a cervical cytology test is payable only for tests carried out on women over the age of 35, who are most at risk, or those under 35 with three or more children. A yearly fee is paid to general practitioners for providing contraceptive services and advice, with a higher fee for fitting intrauterine devices (IUDs). Maternity services attract a fee for the various components of the service, for complete care or for ante- and post-natal care only. There are also fees payable for treating temporary residents, for emergency treatment, and for night visits.

Each fee or allowance is designed to provide approximately two thirds net income and one third expenses with the exception of the designated area allowance, seniority allowance, vocational training allowance, post graduate training allowance, trainers grant and inducement payments, which are considered to be pure net income for superannuation purposes.

Employment of ancillary staff

The system by which general practitioners can employ ancillary staff was improved with the Family Doctor Charter so that most of the costs of employing staff could be borne by the Family Practitioner Committee and not by the practice itself. The practice has a great deal of freedom as an employer, over salary levels and employment conditions. The 70 per cent reimbursement of salaries also covers ancillary staff carrying out other qualifying duties, which are listed as secretarial and clerical, receiving patients, making appointments and dispensing, as well as nursing and treatment. The staff covered include practice managers, secretaries, receptionists, book keepers and dispensers as well as practice nurses. To qualify for the full 70 per cent reimbursement of salaries, a general practitioner must have at least 1000 patients on his or her list and the staff must be employed on a regular basis for at least 5 hours per week. As well as receiving 70 per cent reimbursement of salaries, the doctor also receives reimbursement of national insurance and superannuation costs and 70 per cent of any training costs for the staff members. The remaining 30 per cent staff wages which have to be paid for by the practice are indirectly reimbursed to all general practitioners by way of their gross fees and allowances which are taken into account by the Review Body (Lowe, 1982). The remaining third is also an allowable expense for tax purposes. Practices have wide discretion over staffing levels. They could employ up to two staff members for each partner and get reimbursement. In fact on average, family doctors only employ just over one staff member per doctor. Most practices employ receptionists, but there is much greater variability in the employment of nursing staff.

Employment of nurses

Nursing staff can either be attached to practices or employed directly by them. Attachment is common. About 80 per cent of district nurses and 75 per cent of health visitors are attached to practices. For a long time this arrangement was encouraged but recently it has come under increasing criticism. Research has shown that relationships between family doctors and attached nurses are often poor (Bond *et al*, 1987) and the Cumberlege Report recommended that nursing teams would be better organised on a neighbourhood basis (Department of Health and Social Security, 1986a). The direct employment of nurses by practices was also encouraged for many years. The idea is not a new one and such employment started as early as 1911 (Davidson, 1982). One in four of practices now employ nurses, but the numbers of staff per general practitioner actually employed currently stands at only 1.1 and most of these are receptionists (Hart, 1985). As with attachment there has been recent controversy over the employment of nurses, with recommendations from the Cumberlege Report that reimbursement should cease. (Department of Health and Social Security, 1986a). However the White Paper on primary care (Department of Health and Social Security, 1987) recommended that the ratio of ancillary staff to general practitioners should be increased and restrictions on the type of staff employed under this system be reduced.

Trainers and trainees

The introduction of the vocational training scheme faced practices with further decisions. About 10 per cent of general practitioner principals are now trainers. Trainers were found in one study to have graduated more recently, to subscribe to more journals and to be more likely to use medical libraries than non trainers (Hay *et al*, 1980).

Since February 1981, a doctor has been unable to become a principal without spending a year as a trainee in general practice. The second part of the National Health Service Vocational Training Act 1977 was implemented in August 1982. This required a potential general practitioner to spend two years in hospital approved posts in addition to the year in general practice, making a total of three years' training for general practice. One of the hospital years had to consist of two spells of six months on named specialties, to be selected from accident and emergency or general surgery, general medicine, geriatrics, obstetrics and gynaecology, paediatrics or psychiatry.

The second hospital year offers a wider choice and can be more of the same, or totally different (General Practitioner, 1982). Training can be undertaken on a part-time basis but must be completed within 7 years. Standards of placements are monitored by the Joint Committee for Postgraduate Training in General Practice (JCPTGP) which was created in 1975. It set out standards for medical records which all training practices should attain; hence the concern found in the current study for the organisation of practice records and the various attempts being made to rationalise them.

The JCPTGP has set out a list of criteria for the selection of trainers (JCPTGP, 1980) and all potential trainers are expected to attend a week long course. There is also a practice visit. Approval rates are around 85 per cent, and rejected applicants can appeal. More stringent criteria have been suggested for the selection of trainers (Cameron, 1983).

In terms of raising standards and subjecting practices to an inspection, the trainee scheme has obvious advantages, as well as providing extra assistance in the practice.

The improvement of premises

Before the Family Doctor Charter, general practitioners had virtually no accessible source of funding for improving their premises. The health centre programme had not been a success. New schemes have given the general practitioner much more scope for initiative and there has been a strong response.

1. *Direct reimbursement of rent and rates* The Family Doctor Charter introduced direct reimbursement of rent and rates to general practitioners for their practice premises. The aim was both to reimburse general practitioners against the cost of providing practice premises and to create an incentive to them to maintain their premises in an acceptable condition. Family Practitioner Committees are encouraged to make periodic inspections and withhold payment if premises are considered to be substandard.

Reimbursement of rent is allowed for all general practitioners with more than 100 patients on their list, and consists of direct reimbursement in the case of rented property, notional rent for owner-occupiers, or cost rent reimbursement for purpose-built or improved property.

2. *Notional rent* A notional rent, reviewed every three years, and equivalent to the current market rent, is paid to general practitioners who own their own premises. The rent is assessed by the District Valuer (British Medical Journal, 1977) and agreement can be problematic. In an attempt to smooth out any difficulties, regional panels of surveyors were set up in 1981 to give independent advice to general practitioners and help them to liaise with Family Practitioner Committees (British Medical Journal, 1981). The notional rent usually represents approximately 80 per cent of the resale value of the practice premises. Over 90 per cent of appeals against the reassessment value of rents have been successful in achieving an increase (Lowe, 1982a).

3. *Cost rent* General practitioners financing their practice premises can receive either a notional rent (see above) or a cost rent. Cost rent is available for (a) building completely new premises (b) acquiring and substantially altering premises and (c) substantially altering existing practice premises. The premises may be either owned or rented by the doctor (British Medical Journal, 1977).

The cost rent is made up of (a) the cost or current market value of the site, whichever is less (b) legal and other fees (c) the cost of the building work to the lowest tender, subject to cost limits and (d) interest charges on interim loans. The cost rent is effectively an interest free loan.

General practitioners renting purpose-built premises may also receive a cost rent which is a percentage of (a) the current market value of the site (b) the notional building costs, cost-limited and (c) the legal costs.

The initial cost rent will usually be higher than the notional rent because building costs are often higher than the value of the completed building. The cost rent remains static but notional rents are reassessed every three years in line with increasing property values. It usually becomes advantageous to transfer to notional rent after 6-9 years (Lowe, 1981). Cost rent schemes are usually financed by the General Practice Finance Corporation.

4. *The General Practice Finance Corporation (GPFC)* The General Practice Finance Corporation was set up in 1967 as a result of the Family Doctor Charter. Before this, general practitioners had very little help with the provision of premises since conventional sources of capital tended not to lend for long enough (British Medical Journal, 1979). At that time, the only source of funds specifically for general practitioners was the Group Practice Loans Scheme which was set up in 1954. This scheme had many disadvantages, however, since it would only lend up to 80 per cent of the amount required, and was only available to doctors practising in recognised groups. In addition, the scheme was financed from the central pool from which general practitioners were paid. The scheme was discontinued with the advent of the GPFC.

By 1986 the GPFC had made 4364 loans to 8239 general practitioners for £99.2 million of which £80.5 million was outstanding in 1986 (General Practice Finance Corporation, 1986). GPFC borrowing, net of stock redemption, over the past 5 years has been 1981/82, £4.5m; 1982/3, £3.5m; 1983/4, £12.7m; 1984/5, £23.3m and 1985/6, £22.5m (Department of Health and Social Security, 1986b). The number of loans taken up in Great Britain has fallen by 25 per cent between 1984/5 and 1985/6, but the loans are larger. East Anglia and the South West are the only regions to show an increase in loans taken out in the period. All other regions showed a fall (General Practice Finance Corporation, 1986).

The GPFC has been less successful in developing special incentives for investment in inner city practices. The Acheson report of 1981 spelled out the special problems of practices in such areas (Department of Health and Social Security, 1981). Property is frequently unsuitable for conversion and too expensive to finance. A traditional solution has been the building of health centres, but these tended to be long term enterprises and cannot be the remedy in the short term. In addition, they are frequently unpopular with doctors.

The government has recently outlined plans to privatise the GPFC so that its borrowings will no longer count towards the Public Sector Borrowing Requirement (PSBR). The aim is to reduce the GPFC borrowing by more than half, to £12 million from 1st April 1987 and to less than £5 million per year by 1990. 80 per cent of loans will in future be financed from the private sector. Hambros Bank was appointed to conduct a feasibility study into private financing for surgery premises. The fall in numbers of loans from the GPFC suggests that there has already been some development of private alternatives.

5. *The buy and leaseback scheme* From the start, the GPFC has wanted to be allowed to buy or build premises itself and lease them back to general practitioners. Initially, this was ruled out on the grounds that it would duplicate the health centre building programme. Instead, the GPFC was allowed to lease land to doctors for building premises. This facility was rarely used because the cost of land represents only a very small proportion of the cost of surgery premises. Since April 1981, a buy and lease back scheme has been in existence and has been especially beneficial to inner city doctors who face high land and property prices (Russell, 1981; British Medical Journal, 1981a).

6. *Improvement grants* General practitioners are able, through the Family Practitioner Committee, to make use of improvement grants which can provide 30 per cent of the cost of smaller alterations such as extensions, internal improvements and the provision of car parks (Lowe, 1981a). Grants of up to 60 per cent are available for premises not previously used as practice premises in certain areas, but new buildings are not eligible (Hall, 1986). General practitioners have to find the outstanding amount of money from other sources, and do their own decorations and repairs. The grants can be helpful for inner city doctors where sites for new premises are either too expensive or not readily available, but take up has been patchy. Some urban areas have had very few schemes while in Cheshire 72 per cent of all premises have been improved. (Allsop and May, 1986).

7. *Health centres* General practitioners can also rent premises. Rented property consists mainly of health centres which are owned by the District Health Authority and rented to family doctors. More rarely, property can be privately rented. Health centre building increased sharply in the 1970s but has since fallen from favour and the private provision of premises has become more popular, particularly by making use of the cost rent scheme.

Doctors working from health centres have certain advantages in that other health services and clinics may be available to them and their patients in the same building: yet these doctors are more constrained by space and frequently complain that they would like to expand their services but are unable to do so because of lack of space. Doctors who purchase their own premises may have to spend more of their practice profits on paying off loans while they are in practice; but they benefit from the sale of their share of the premises on retirement. By contrast, young doctors entering general practice may face financial difficulties in buying into privately owned practice premises, whereas health centre doctors do not have such problems. It was envisaged at the beginning of the National Health Service that the health centre programme would be the main way of improving premises for family doctors. Little was heard of the programme for many years. It became active from 1966 to 1979 when health centre numbers increased from 212 to 929, but, since then, few health centres have been built. Even so, in England today, one doctor in five works in a health centre and in Northern Ireland the proportion is 54 per cent.

Equipment levels in general practice

At the present time, there is little financial incentive for family doctors to invest in practice equipment other than a few basic items. The incentives to do so come mainly from increased professional satisfaction and from being able to provide a better service for patients.

This investigation has attempted to discover what equipment is owned by the family doctors in the study areas, and also to find out what equipment they would like to have, but it is important, initially, to set out the context in which the medical equipment industry operates. Equipment levels in general practice are also affected by the degree of access to hospital based laboratory services, and this has, in part, contributed to the limited technological development in general practice.

There is cheap and easy to manipulate equipment available to general practitioners in the United Kingdom. Such equipment is widely used by physicians in the United States of America and in other European countries, but British family doctors have been slow to make use of it (Kuenssberg, 1980). The technology now exists to carry out diagnostic tests using kits which perform the tests at the touch of a button. It is no longer necessary to use bottles of reagents which have to be made up by technical assistants who are responsible for calibration and standardisation. General practitioners could in principle do these tests, but in Great Britain this is usually left to hospitals, via open access. The system does, however, avoid the major problem of servicing and testing for accuracy of many small, scattered units (Kuenssberg, 1980). Practices carrying out their own tests might be popular with patients who bear the hidden costs of travel to hospital and time taken for tests. In addition, results would be available immediately and the appropriate treatment could be started at once.

A problem with tests is the current lack of expertise in their use by general practitioners, and the problems of standardisation. The equipment would need regular calibration with the local hospital, which would still be responsible for the bulk of diagnostic tests, performed on their own patients. Although general practitioners' requests to hospital laboratories for diagnostic tests have steadily increased, these requests still form only about 10 per cent of the total laboratory workload. In the past it was much more efficient for tests to be centralised and this centralisation has been the main reason why general practitioners have not performed their own tests.

Any general practitioner currently investing in diagnostic equipment would have to finance the basic equipment and associated consumables. The benefit might be felt in increased professional and patient satisfaction but there are considerable financial disincentives. Although 70 per cent of staffing costs are reimbursed to general practitioners, such reimbursement does not apply to equipment costs. Spending on equipment can currently only be recouped if it enables the family doctor to support more patients or provide special services for which an "item of service" payment is made.

One suggestion made in the White Paper (Department of Health and Social Security, 1987) is that general practitioners should provide a wide range of preventive services to patients. Service targets could be defined for particular groups such as blood pressure checks for over 45s and glucose checks on diabetics, and there could be rewards for achieving these targets. If test facilities were available on the general practitioners' premises, then these services would be likely to be provided. A report by ACARD, (ACARD, 1986) concerned with the medical equipment industry in the United Kingdom, recommended that the family doctor expenses system should be revised to encourage the purchase of equipment. Such a development might help to reduce hospital admissions (Michael, 1981).

Computers in general practice

In contrast to the detailed commitment on policies aimed at improving premises, the Family Doctor Charter had little to say about improving working capital and equipment. However, in the 1980s, change in technology brought such issues more to the fore.

Since the late 1970s, micro-computers have become cheap and accessible. The implications for general practitioners were described in the Royal College of General Practitioner's report of the computer working party (Royal College of General Practitioners, 1980), and in the Scicon Report (Palmer and Rees, 1980) commissioned by the General Medical Services Committee of the British Medical Association, which favoured the phased introduction of computers for general practitioners (Ritchie, 1982). In 1980, a Joint Policy Group comprising members of the Computer Working Party and the British Medical Association was set up, and two years later reported to the Department of Health and Social Security in the document "Computers in Primary Care" (Royal College of General Practitioners, 1982). These reports led to the implementation of the "micros for GPs" scheme in 1982.

In June of the same year, the Government announced it would make available £2.5m for the development and purchase of computers for general practitioners and Family Practitioner Committees. The Government would finance the major part of the purchase, installation costs and maintenance for three years, of 150 computers for general practitioners in the United Kingdom, with any remaining costs being met by the practices concerned (Hansard, 1982). It would finance the Family Practitioner Committee part of the project which would cost £1m and give two Family Practitioner Committees computation facilities for patient registration, and set up cervical cytology call and recall schemes for 20 Family Practitioner Committees. The remaining £1.5m would be for the "micros for GPs" scheme. The scheme was designed to provide evidence on the costs and difficulties of introducing computers, the reliability of the systems installed, the attitudes of staff and users, safety and efficiency, benefits to patients and effects on practice administration. (Chinque, 1984).

1015 practices expressed an initial interest in the "micros for GPs" scheme and 850 practices subsequently applied for a system. By 1984, 150 practices had been selected to take part. Distribution of computers was to be spread around the country, with regional coordinators in each area. Regional coordinators would receive a free computer for their own practice and a fee for their work (Nenk, 1982). As a condition of receiving a computer, practices were asked to take part in an evaluation exercise, and the results were thought likely to be of some general interest to family doctors. (Stoddart, 1984).A small number of practices were to be studied in depth (Department of Health and Social Security, 1984).

The practices chosen to take part in the study would face average costs of £7000 over 3 years, which could be set against tax. Staffing was paid for by an allowance of 10-20p per record transferred to the computer. There was criticism that only two companies were selected to supply computers for the scheme and fears that smaller companies would be unable to compete, but this did not happen. Although two or three companies did withdraw from the family doctors market, the market, as a whole, has remained extensive with about 40 companies in the field (Jessop, 1984). However, in 1984, only half of computerised practices were in the scheme at all with the remaining practices using more than 30 different computing systems (Stoddart, 1984).

In 1985, the Department of Health and Social Security produced the final report on the scheme, comparing practices with and without computers (Department of Health and Social Security, 1985) together with further reports (Department of Health and Social Security 1986c and d) on the longer term potential of computers in general practice. The computerised practices had now had computers for at least 2 years. It was noted that considerable initial effort was required to computerise, and concluded that as many staff as possible should take part in the process. Once the initial teething problems were over, most practices felt they would keep their computer. Computers were found to create more work, but they did allow practices to operate more efficiently or to expand the range of work done. However the scheme showed how difficult it would be to develop incentives for the use of working capital which could be as effective as those for improving premises had proved to be.

A fourth phase

The Family Doctor Charter in essence represented a considerable step forward from the previous half century. Many of the policy aims which it set were achieved. It led to much improved recruitment, helped by a shift in career preferences in favour of general practice. It also accelerated the movement towards larger practices so that by 1986, 52 per cent of family doctors were working in practices with four or more partners. Investment in premises was encouraged so that by 1986 many practices were working in new or improved premises. The Family Doctor Charter stimulated the employment of ancillary staff although the effectiveness of these changes in promoting real team work remained a subject of debate. It encouraged the development of vocational training and provided a financial basis for the training system.

Previously there had been conflict between the Ministry of Health's interest in cost containment and the desire of general practitioners to preserve their independent contractor status. Under the original Family Doctor Charter, there was more local discretion allowing different strategies by practices in employment of staff and investment in premises. The changes and additions to the Charter since 1965 have strengthened these discretionary elements. The fee for service element has been expanded and the financing of new premises has gradually been privatised so that it is now the responsibility of the partnership to make the best deal open to it in an independent way. The new programme for encouraging the use of computers is a further example of a discretionary policy.

By the mid-1980s there seemed to be greater awareness of the deficiencies of the Family Doctor Charter. The most usual critique (and that set out by the Department of Health and Social Security (Department of Health and Social Security, 1986)) stressed the variability in standard of services. Other common complaints were about insufficient choice for patients, the blocking of primary care teamwork and the perversity of the payment system which rewarded inertia rather than active or preventive care. (Royal College of General Practitioners, 1985). General practice seemed to be entering a fourth phase. What would seem to be the critical issues in this phase?

The evidence from the three main phases in the development of general practice - the panel doctor system and the two stages of development within the National Health Service - showed the continuity of the same issues. In each period, the central issues have been those of income levels, recruitment to general practice and professional status; issues on the supply side. Questions concerned with service quality and the demand for services have been raised but have not led to any clear action. Under the panel system there were complaints about the standard of maternity care and about the treatment of fractures. (Honigsbaum, 1979). Early in the life of the National Health Service there were complaints about the standard of care in urban general practice (Collings, 1950) and later under the Family Doctor Charter there were criticisms of the six minute consultation and of the inconsistency in service quality between practices. (Cartwright and Anderson, 1981).

One characteristic of the fourth phase is that issues of service quality and of the pattern of demand have become much more central to the discussion (Butler and Calnan, 1987). For the first time there is a serious possibility of change within the system even though the current state of pay and manpower is causing no more than routine concern. The fourth phase could be seen in terms of consumerism and the demand for more information by patients, but change is likely to be slow so long as patients remain deferential. A more important feature of the fourth period will be the shift of professional focus from inputs towards outputs, with new concerns about the quality of output and its cost. The relative costs of different programmes in primary and out-patient care have begun to attract attention.

For three decades after 1945, the expansion of health services in developed countries concentrated on hospital services, where all the resources of high technology medicine were brought to bear on the cure of disease. Primary care was considered a second best, mainly for developing countries. Even in Britain, primary care was to be shaped as closely as possible to the model of hospital care, through the building of larger health centres. Since the mid 1970s, there has been a loss of confidence in the model and increased criticism of the effectiveness of hospital care.

The most constructive and influential response so far has been from the World Health Organisation (World Health Organisation, 1978). The Alma Ata declaration outlined an alternative model of health services. The declaration saw primary health care as the main way forward. It "...addressed...the main health problems in the community, providing preventive, curative, and rehabilitative services accordingly." It aims to give locally accessible services in treatment and prevention, and to work through other government agencies to promote better health; for example, through incentives to reduce smoking. Primary care on this model will try to get local communities and individuals involved in planning and developing services, and will lead to a re-appraisal of the health team to give a greater role to nurses.

Within Britain there has been some increased interest in prevention as a means of reaching the World Health Organisation's Health Targets (Fry and Hasler, 1986). In principle, primary care, as well as providing an entry, screening and referral point for the rest of the health care system, could also assume responsibility for health maintenance and for preventive programmes covering whole populations. Fowler (Fowler, 1986) has argued that primary care is in a unique situation in relation to prevention because of its extensive access to the whole population (Fry and Hasler, 1986).

The Alma Ata Declaration pointed towards a wider approach to primary care going beyond general practice, and it has had an international impact. Within Britain it has become merged with another movement of opinion and research of more domestic origins, which has led to greater criticism of the quality of medical care. It has come to be accepted that Britain's record in mortality and morbidity is poor, with higher levels of preventable disease such as measles and rubella (OECD, 1987). Levels of cervical cancer and breast cancer have remained static or risen, and Britain has one of the highest death rates from heart disease in the developed world. (Office of Health Economics, 1987). There have also been more specific criticisms of the quality of care provided in primary care for people with long-term illness (Kurji and Haines, 1984).

All this criticism has been summed up in terms of an "inconsistency" in general practice, as implied in the following statement from the Royal College of General Practitioners (Royal College of General Practitioners, 1985).

> "Towards one end of the spectrum there is comprehensive care of high quality provided by general practitioners and other members of the primary care team. At the other there is care of such poor quality that patients often seek primary care through hospital accident and emergency departments and specialists continue to manage patients who could be returned to the care of their own doctors."

The problems of achieving consistency in quality are even greater because of variations in workload between areas. In 1975 there was little difference in consultation rates at the regional level. From 1975 to 1986 the position changed so that consultation rates fell or remained unchanged in the South East and East Anglia, while rising sharply over most of the North and the Midlands. The range is now from 3.1 consultations per head per year in East Anglia to 5.1 consultations in Wales, which would mean a difference of 65 per cent in numbers of consultations generated in a year for practices with similar list sizes. (Office of Health Economics, 1987).

Family doctors have changed under the Family Doctor Charter to a system of work with new types of enterprise and higher levels of resources than were found in general practice prior to the Charter. There are now a number of choices on which they have discretion. The response at the level of the individual practice is equally as important as the national system of incentives. In essence family doctors have already started to act as economic agents within an internal market.

The next chapters look at the survey evidence on how family doctors have responded to these new challenges.

3 The methods used in the study

Family doctors work within a set of rules and policies set nationally, but little is known about the adjustment to these at the local level. Practices make decisions on premises, staffing, equipment and the size of partnership but the variation in different parts of the country is not known. There have been studies of clinical decisions such as that of referral to out-patients (Dowie, 1983), but there is little economic evidence on levels of income or cost and resource use on a small area basis. Other studies have tended to concentrate on patients' experience rather than doctors'. (Metcalfe *et al*, 1983).

One reason why there is so little evidence on a small area basis is the extreme difficulty of collecting data from doctors, especially on income and costs. This difficulty has ruled out a national questionnaire on a postal basis. An alternative approach is by direct interview on a small area basis and it is this method which has been adopted here. It should be stressed that the sample is not a national one and cannot be aggregated into one. However the areas were chosen to represent different social and environmental types within England.

The survey of general practice was carried out in a total of 7 separate and distinct Family Practitioner Committee areas in England. The survey aimed to test three hypotheses:

(a) that there would be a differential and consistent response to professional and economic incentives

(b) that the response would be affected by the type of or changes in the local population

(c) that practices which had made the greatest attempt to develop and improve their services would face the greatest financial pressure. Practices make choices and economic decisions about resources such as staffing, equipment and premises and these could be expected to reflect the location of the practice, in particular the social and economic characteristics of the local community.

Methods

1. *The pilot study* This was carried out in Spring 1986, in a single Family Practitioner Committee area in a mining region in the North of England, on the edge of the Pennines. The area consisted of one large town and numerous smaller towns and satellite villages. There were 37 practices, comprising 106 family doctors. The Family Practitioner Committee and Local Medical Committee were informed of the intention to carry out the study and their approval was granted.

Initially, a letter outlining the study was sent to the senior partner in each practice indicating that a researcher would be in touch by telephone to arrange a mutually convenient time for an interview lasting some 30 minutes. Twenty-nine of the 37 practices agreed to an interview, which frequently took longer than the suggested 30 minutes because of the interest shown by the doctors. A "group practice questionnaire" was used for the interviews with the doctors from the 25 group practices, and the four single-handed doctors responded to the necessarily longer "single handed GP questionnaire". Interviews were conducted personally by the authors. At the time of the interview with the doctor in his surgery, an individual questionnaire for each partner in the practice was left for self completion. Each was presented in an individual envelope addressed personally to each doctor, and inside was a stamped-addressed return envelope, the individual GP questionnaire and a personally addressed explanatory letter. The doctor was asked to return the questionnaire within two weeks. Two reminders were sent, and if there was no response, no further action was taken and these doctors were the non responders. Group and individual questionnaires were posted to those doctors who could not be contacted by telephone, or who were unsure. Two responded by post. Personal thank you letters were sent to all responders. Each questionnaire had a code number by which each practice and doctor could be identified only by the researchers.

The questionnaires were analysed by computer and the results are included with the results of the main survey, where appropriate. The single handed doctors were excluded from the analysis and were not interviewed in the main study.

The pilot study achieved an 86 per cent response rate for the personal interview, and a 55 per cent response rate for the postal questionnaire (Bosanquet and Leese, 1986).

2. *Modifications adopted in the methodology for the main study* The pilot study was carried out in order to assess the viability of the methods for the main study. As a result of response rates in the pilot study, a slightly different method was adopted for the main study.

In the pilot study, only 4 (50 per cent) of the eight single handed doctors responded. It was felt that these doctors represented a distinct and declining sub group within the general population and were excluded from the study. The 50 per cent response rate was not considered good enough, though such doctors could merit a separate study at a later date.

Although a 55 per cent response rate had been achieved with the postal questionnaire, this was considered to be inadequate for the main study. It was also found that most doctors, having agreed to an interview, were very happy to talk at length about their practices, and that the interview questionnaire could therefore be lengthened. For the main study, the postal questionnaire was discontinued and the questions, where possible, were included in a slightly longer questionnaire, to be used to interview one partner in each practice. As a result of this policy, some data collected in the pilot study are not directly comparable with those collected in the main study, but, wherever possible, pilot study data have been included in the results of the main study.

The main study

The aim was to collect information from all practices, except the single-handed ones, in all the chosen areas. In two of the six areas, the survey covered the entire Family Practitioner Committee area. In the other four which were very large, the survey covered a large and self-contained part of it. The numbers of practices sampled were similar in all areas. Interviews were carried out in the six selected areas, between October 1986 and May 1987. Family Practitioner Committee listings of family doctors were used, and the agreement of the Local Medical Committee was obtained in all cases. The interviews were carried out by locally recruited interviewers, together with the study authors. The chosen areas, and their characteristics, are listed below.

Area 1: North West Suburban This area has two sizable towns with some light industry and engineering, together with numerous small villages.

Area 2: London Inner City This area has a high proportion of its population from ethnic minorities and has a long experience of deprivation. It is completely urban and has wards which are among the poorest in England.

Area 3: Thames Valley A comparatively affluent area with many smaller towns, but also including a new town and some areas of older urban deprivation.

Area 4: East Rural There is one larger town, several small market towns and some seaside resorts.

Area 5: North East Industrial This area includes three large towns and some villages. It is dependent on heavy manufacturing industry and unemployment is high.

Area 6: Midlands Urban This is a mixed urban area on the edge of a much larger conurbation. It includes a high proportion of its population from ethnic minorities. There is a large amount of council housing, but there are also some more affluent villages.

Area 7: North Mining This is the pilot study area. It is made up of a medium sized town and its environs on the edge of the Pennines. It has a central core, working class estates, some suburban housing developments and many small villages. It is self contained, and at some distance from other towns or cities.

These areas were chosen after examination of research done by the Office of Population Censuses and Surveys on the distribution of the population of England between rural and urban areas (Denham, 1984). The population, and some social characteristics of the chosen areas are given in Table 3.1. Possibly the most significant indicators are the unemployment rate and the degree of overcrowding. Four areas rank from 1 to 4 for both indicators. These are London Inner City, North East Industrial, Midlands Urban and North Mining. These four areas together are less affluent. The other three areas; NW Suburban, Thames Valley and East Rural, form the more affluent group. The areas covered are representative of those in which the great majority of people in England live.

Letters explaining the study were sent to one partner in each practice in the Family Practitioner Committee listings for the chosen areas. This was followed by a telephone call from the interviewer to arrange an interview date. The interview was conducted by the interviewer, usually in the doctor's surgery and was scheduled to take 45 minutes. In the event, many interviews took longer than this as many doctors set out their views on general practice at some length. Local advice was taken on which partner might be interested in taking part in the study. If this partner refused, another was approached. Most practices were extremely helpful and cooperative.

Response rates

Table 3.2 sets out the response rates for each of the seven study areas. The overall response rate was 73 per cent, which compares favourably with the responses achieved in other surveys of general practice. The study of workload carried out by the Review Body in 1986, with the endorsement and support of the British Medical Association and the Department of Health and Social Security achieved a response of only 58 per cent (Department of Health and Social Security, 1987b). The earlier surveys by Cartwright and Anderson had response rates of 76 per cent in 1964 and 67 per cent in 1977 (Cartwright, 1967 and Cartwright and Anderson, 1981) and Butler and Calnan achieved a response rate of 67 per cent (Butler and Calnan, 1987).

The response rate was poorest in Area 2 (London Inner City). Even after many more telephone calls than were necessary in other areas, the response rate still only reached 64 per cent. In other areas, there is no reason to think that the survey was biased in particular directions. However, within Area 2, it may well be that the survey covered more of the innovatory practices, and this factor will be considered when discussing the survey results. Cartwright and Anderson had experienced particular problems in achieving a response from practices with Asian doctors (Cartwright and Anderson, 1981). The results where there was a high percentage of Asian general practitioners suggest there might be a reluctance on the part of these doctors, working under particularly difficult circumstances, to take part in surveys.

In Area 7, the pilot study area, there was a total of 87 doctors in all the responding practices, but only 52 completed the individual doctor questionnaire. Table 3.3 gives some information on the responding and non-responding practices.

Table 3.1
Selected social characteristics of study areas

	(1) NW Suburban	(2) London Inner City	(3) Thames Valley	(4) East Rural	(5) NE Industrial	(6) Midlands Urban	(7) North Mining
Total res. pop	436,354	251,238	307,185	485,350	565,845	550,986	223,903
% 65+	13.9	13.2	11.8	17.8	11.3	13.2	13.5
% under 5s	5.6	6.3	6.6	5.5	6.8	6.1	5.8
Unemployed as % of population 16-65	8.6	10.2	5.7	7.7	16.9	14.0	10.5
Rank	(5)	(4)	(7)	(6)	(1)	(2)	(3)
Overcrowded households as % of total	4.4	17.2	7.3	3.7	8.4	10.2	8.1
Rank	(6)	(1)	(5)	(7)	(3)	(2)	(4)
1 parent families as % of total households	1.4	3.1	1.8	1.4	2.3	1.9	1.8
Unskilled as % of population 16-65	3.7	4.4	3.0	3.2	7.4	4.6	3.9
Households lacking amenity as % of total	3.2	5.5	3.1	3.3	3.0	5.0	2.3
Households from ethnic minorities as % of total	0.8	33.2	7.7	0.7	1.6	10.1	0.4

Source: Office of Population, Censuses and Surveys, 1983.

Table 3.2
Response rates by area

Area	% Response	Number of responding partnerships	Total number of partnerships	Total number of practices	Single handed % of total
7. North Mining	86	25	29	37	22
1. NW Suburban	80	41	51	59	14
4. East Rural	74	40	54	65	17
5. NE Industrial	72	47	65	82	21
3. Thames Valley	70	32	46	58	21
6. Midlands Urban	70	48	69	127	46
2. London Inner City	64	27	42	91	54
Total	73	260	356	519	31

Some information on respondents is set out in Table 3.4 which shows that response rates were lower among two partner practices.

Single handed general practitioners were excluded from the study, but some characteristics of this group in each of the study areas have been collected and are shown in Table 3.5. Most of the single handed general practitioners were practising in urban areas which together contained 66 per cent of all the single handed doctors in the 7 areas. Most of these doctors (91 per cent) were male, and 52 per cent were Asian. The non-Asian doctors tended to be older than the average for all the single handed doctors, confirming the often stated view that single handed doctors in inner city areas are often elderly. The average age of all the single handed doctors was 49 years, but that of the non Asians was 53 years. These figures should be compared with the average of 44 years for all doctors in partnerships, and for single handed Asians of 45 years. Single handed practice therefore remains of great significance in the urban areas such as London Inner City and Midlands Urban, but less so in other, more rural or suburban areas. 52 per cent of the single handed general practitioners in all of the urban areas were Asian but this ranged from 72 per cent in Area 6 (Midlands Urban) to only 18 per cent in Area 4 (East Rural), confirming the concentration of Asian general practitioners in urban areas.

Table 3.3
Some characteristics of responding and non-responding doctors

Area	Respondents as % of all doctors	Number of doctors in responding practices	Number of doctors in non responding practices	Total number of doctors	Number of Asian non-responders	Number of non-Asian non responders
North Mining	90	87	10	97	10	0
NW Suburban	82	172	38	210	1	37
East Rural	79	159	43	202	2	41
NE Industrial	79	193	50	243	9	41
Thames Valley	73	127	48	175	6	42
Midlands Urban	73	149	54	203	23	31
London Inner City	70	83	35	118	15	20
Total	78	970	278	1248	66	212

Table 3.4
Percentage response by area and size of practice

Area	Partnership size 2	3	4	5	6	7+
1. NW Suburban	87	70	67	91	89	100
2. North Mining	80	86	86	100	-	100
3. Thames Valley	56	78	75	67	100	100
6. Midlands Urban	55	76	73	100	-	-
4. East Rural	54	72	90	67	100	75
2. London Inner City	52	69	100	100	100	100
5. NE Industrial	50	78	100	60	100	100

Table 3.5
Characteristics of the single-handed doctors by study area

	(6) Midlands Urban	(2) London Inner City	(5) NE Industrial	(3) Thames Valley	(4) East Rural	(1) NW Suburban	(7) North Mining	Total
No. single-handed doctors	58	49	17	12	11	8	8	163
No. female doctors (%)	2 (3)	11 (22)	0 (0)	1 (8)	0 (0)	0 (0)	1 (13)	15 (9)
No. Asian doctors (%)	42 (72)	21 (43)	5 (29)	7 (58)	2 (18)	2 (25)	5 (63)	84 (52)
Age (years)								
Average age of all single-handed	50	55	43	41	51	50	51	49
Average age of all Asian single-handed	47	49	43	46	40	39	49	45
Average age of all non-Asian single-handed	57	57	43	49	54	54	54	53
% Single-handed GPs								
aged under 50	55	51	89	82	45	50	38	57
aged 51-59	24	22	12	18	36	13	50	23
aged over 60	21	27	0	0	18	38	13	19
No. Asians aged over 60	1	1	0	0	0	0	0	2

Conclusions

The research problem was that of assessing a situation where the usual option of a national questionnaire survey was not possible. On a postal basis the response would have been poor while on an interview basis such a survey would have been too expensive. A number of representative areas were therefore chosen and all practices in the areas were approached for interview. The areas formed either the whole of a small Family Practitioner Committee area or a self-contained sub-division of a larger one. In all cases the areas were large enough to form self-contained medical "markets". A standard questionnaire was piloted and interviewers selected. A good response was achieved as a result of the ready co-operation of many practices. Overall, data were collected from a total of 260 practices and 970 family doctors in the seven areas.

The research method adopted allows more testing of hypotheses about the effects of local environment as against personal characteristics than would have been possible with a national questionnaire. The model used (see Figure 1.1) relates these factors to decisions on practice structure and to outcomes for doctors. On a small area basis it was easier to relate all these variables in a consistent way. The method adopted may have been enforced by cost and response problems, but it also suited the aims of the study.

4 Local variations

Chapter 1 presented a review of aggregate national data on practice structure. This chapter presents the data from the survey which show the variation in the pattern of practice organisation among the 7 study areas.

Succeeding chapters deal more fully with the causation of these differences, and with outcomes for the doctors and for the patients. This chapter establishes the extent of variations in practice decisions in relation to the personal characteristics of the doctors, the payment system, the practice location and local environment, as shown in Figure 1.1 and in Table 1.8.

General practitioner characteristics

1. *Age* Data have been collected on the age of the individual doctors from which it has been possible to calculate the average age of the doctors in each study area. The age variable could have been defined in a number of ways. The data were collected as the ages of the individual doctors and it was necessary to relate this information to each practice and area as a whole to facilitate analysis. Age bands could have been used, but it was decided to use this approach only to define the numbers of practices with an average age of the partners of over 50 years, as shown in Table 4.1. Although average age is an imperfect variable since it hides the many possible age structures within a practice or area, it was considered to be the most appropriate way of presenting the results. These reservations should, however, be borne in mind. Table 4.1 indicates that there was little variation in average age between areas.

Table 4.1
Average age of partners by area

Area	Average age of partners (years)	Practices where average average age of partner is over 50 years %	no	Total no. of practices
2. London Inner City	46.2	26	(7)	27
6. Midlands Urban	44.7	21	(10)	48
3. Thames Valley	43.9	13	(4)	32
1. NW Suburban	43.4	12	(5)	41
4. East Rural	43.1	3	(1)	40
7. North Mining	43.0	20	(5)	25
5. NE Industrial	42.2	4	(2)	47

However, the average conceals more significant variations in the numbers of practices where the average age of the partners is over 50 years. In three areas, London Inner City (Area 2), Midlands Urban (Area 6) and North Mining (Area 7), the average age of the partnerships was greater than 50 years in at least 20 per cent of the practices.

There was a certain amount of criticism of the rigidity of attitude of older doctors by some younger ones: "Suspect the atmosphere will change when Dr ... retires", "Taken over three elderly practices and forcing them into the 20th Century", "I would like changes - but the senior partner would not". However, such views were not only confined to the younger doctors. One older doctor remarked, "My junior partners may wish to make some changes", and another made the point that his answers may not be truly representative of the views of the other younger doctors. The situation can be summed up by the comment of one interviewer: "There are many examples where the younger partner wants to bring about changes but is not getting support for his ideas".

2. *Sex* The aggregate data set out in Table 1.6 show that nationally the proportions of female general practitioners have been increasing. In the study areas, the proportions of female partners were similar in 4 of the areas, but were much higher in Area 2 (London Inner City) and lower in Area 4 (East Rural). The overall figure of 17 per cent of partners being female compares with the figure for England of 20 per cent in 1984 (Department of Health and Social Security, 1987a). Table 4.2 shows the percentages of female partners in each of the study areas.

Table 4.2
The distribution of female partners by area

Area	Practices with at least 1 female partner %	no	Female doctors in each area %	no
2. London Inner City	70	(19)	37	(31)
1. NW Suburban	66	(27)	17	(30)
3. Thames Valley	63	(20)	22	(28)
5. NE Industrial	51	(24)	15	(29)
6. Midlands Urban	44	(21)	17	(25)
7. North Mining	32	(8)	13	(12)
4. East Rural	30	(12)	8	(12)
Total	50	(131)	17	(167)

Table 4.3
The distribution of Asian partners by area

Area	Practices with at least 1 Asian partner %	no	Asian doctors in each area %	no
7. North Mining	60	(15)	35	(30)
6. Midlands Urban	42	(20)	21	(31)
5. NE Industrial	40	(19)	14	(26)
2. London Inner City	37	(10)	18	(15)
3. Thames Valley	16	(5)	8	(10)
1. NW Suburban	12	(5)	5	(8)
4. East Rural	3	(1)	1	(1)
Total	29	(75)	13	(121)

3. *Ethnic background* In all 7 study areas, a total of 121 (13 per cent) of the doctors were of Asian origin. 102 of these (84 per cent) were working in practices in urban areas (Areas 2, 5, 6 and 7) whereas the more affluent areas (Areas 1, 3 and 4) had only 19 (16 per cent) of the Asian general practitioners (Table 4.3).

4. *Length of service* There was little difference in the average time family doctors had been in their present practice (Table 4.4).

Table 4.4
Average time spent in their present practice, by area

Area	Average no. of years in present practice
1. NW Suburban	13
2. London Inner City	14
3. Thames Valley	13
4. East Rural	12
5. NE Industrial	13
6. Midlands Urban	14
7. North Mining	11

5. *The nature of the contract* The data in Table 4.5 show that the proportions of practices with part-time partners varied greatly between areas. Of the 95 part-time doctors in 6 of the areas (data were not collected for Area 7), 59 (62 per cent) were female and had an average age of 36.4 years. By contrast, the 36 part-time male doctors had an average age of 59.1 years. The general trend was therefore for the female part-time doctors to be younger and the male part-timers to be older, often having taken twenty-four hour retirement. There were a few exceptions to this rule with five part-time female doctors being over 50 years of age, and five part-time males being under 45 years of age. Area 2 (London Inner City) was unique in having ten part-timers, of whom three were males under the age of 41 and two were females of 58 and 60 years. Overall, whereas only 5 per cent of male doctors were part-time, 38 per cent of female doctors worked on a part-time basis (Table 4.5).

Family doctors on part-time contracts were made up of two distinct and dissimilar groups. They were either older male part-timers, of whom there were some in all areas, or they were younger female doctors, who were most common in three areas (1, 3 and 5) two of which were among the more affluent study areas.

6. *Membership of professional organisations* There were some differences between areas in membership of the British Medical Association although the membership level was at least 60 per cent in all areas. BMA membership was higher in the less affluent areas (North East Industrial, London Inner City, North Mining and Midlands Urban). Membership levels in the RCGP were on average much lower than the BMA

and were 40 per cent or more in only two areas (North East Industrial and London Inner City)(Table 4.6).

Table 4.5
The distribution of part-time partners by area

Area	Practices with at least one part-time partner %	no	*Female part-time partners %	no	*Male part-time partners %	no
1. NW Suburban	54	(22)	53	(16)	8	(11)
5. NE Industrial	49	(23)	48	(14)	8	(13)
3. Thames Valley	38	(12)	46	(13)	2	(2)
2. London Inner City	30	(8)	19	(6)	8	(4)
4. East Rural	23	(9)	50	(6)	2	(3)
6. Midlands Urban	15	(7)	16	(4)	2	(3)
Total	35	(81)	35	(59)	5	(36)

* % of female/male doctors in that area who work part-time.

Table 4.6
Membership of RCGP and BMA, by area

Area	Doctors in RCGP %	no	Doctors in BMA %	no	Total number of doctors
5. NE Industrial	45	(86)	78	(150)	193
2. London Inner City	40	(33)	86	(71)	83
3. Thames Valley	34	(43)	69	(88)	127
7. North Mining	31	(16)	81	(42)	52*
1. NW Suburban	30	(52)	60	(103)	172
4. East Rural	27	(43)	64	(102)	159
6. Midlands Urban	27	(40)	75	(112)	149
Total	33	(313)	71	(668)	935

* 52 doctors out of the 87 in Area 7 respondedto the individual general practitioner questionnaire in the pilot study.

7. *Outside posts* Many doctors held posts outside general practice (Table 4.7). Such posts ranged from medical assistantships in a local hospital, to locum work, medical officers for companies etc. Overall, 78 per cent of practices in Areas 1-6 had at least one partner who had at least one post (however small) outside of the practice. Differences were small between areas, although the comparatively smaller number of practices in Area 4 with partners with outside posts may be a reflection of higher incomes and income from dispensing in this area. In other words, they were less likely to wish or need to augment their income. Similar information was collected for individual doctors in Area 7 (North Mining). Here, 18 (35 per cent) of the doctors had outside posts, fewer than in the other 6 areas.

Table 4.7
Practices in which at least one partner had outside post(s), by area

	Practices with at least one partner with outside posts	
Area	%	no
3. Thames Valley	88	(28)
1. NW Suburban	85	(35)
5. NE Industrial	83	(39)
2. London Inner City	78	(21)
6. Midlands Urban	73	(35)
4. East Rural	65	(26)
Total	78	(184)

The payments system

In principle, there would seem to be one single national system of payment, which has been described in detail in Chapter 2. However, local conditions may affect the level of income achieved by practices, as will be shown in Chapter 6. For example, income varies with list size, because of capitation payments, but list size may vary with local demography. Areas with rising populations might be expected to have rising list sizes, but there are other reasons for changes in list size which might offset these demographic effects. List size might vary with the age of practitioners. As doctors got older they might be unwilling to take on new patients and list size would show a gradual decline. List size might also vary with practice strategy, as certain types of practice try to increase their patient numbers.

As Table 4.8 shows, the payment system interacting with other variables can produce wide differences in achieved net income per partner.

Differences were such that net income at the lower quartile in the Thames Valley and East Rural areas was greater than the median value in the Midlands Urban area. The Review Body deals with aggregates and averages but the local reality is that of much greater variability.

Table 4.8
Differences in net income per partner, by area (£,000)

Area	Lower quartile	Median	Upper quartile	Coefficient of variation*
1. NW Suburban	22.7	26.0	30.0	20.5
2. London Inner City	20.0	23.3	28.0	26.6
3. Thames Valley	24.2	28.3	34.7	27.6
4. East Rural	30.0	33.9	37.7	23.1
5. NE Industrial	23.3	26.7	32.3	23.2
6. Midlands Urban	17.5	23.3	28.3	29.2

*Standard deviation as a percentage of the mean.

Practice location and local environment

1. *Social characteristics of the area* The local environment can affect practice decisions in a number of ways. Different attitudes by patients could produce varying degrees of pressure on practices to improve services. There might be more pressure on practices in affluent areas to provide new services and to improve premises, reflecting changes in the local environment. These affluent areas will often be ones in which population will be rising with new housing developments. Opportunities will arise to increase partnership or list size, and for increased partnership income. Such effects may lead to differences within areas as well as between areas since there are affluent parts even in the poorer areas of the survey.

Practices are taking decisions against a background of shifts in population and of greater variability in the local environment. The recent and continuing rapid development of private sector housing has been one factor in operation. Another has been the problem of maintenance of local authority housing. The survey of social attitudes in Britain (Jowell and Airey, 1984) has shown that 84 per cent of owner occupiers thought their local environment had either stayed the same or improved in the last two years, but that 41 per cent of council tenants thought that council estates were unpleasant places in which to live. Patterns of settlement have changed. Data from the Office of Population Censuses and Surveys (Denham, 1984) have recorded population decline in many northern industrial towns and population increases in suburban areas, especially in the south of England. By 1981, there were already more people living in the Aldershot/Bracknell urban area than in Sunderland, and more people in the South coast "conurbation" between Brighton and Bournemouth than in Tyneside and Teesside put together (Denham, 1984).

2. *Changes in the local population* The local impact of some of these changes can be seen in the seven study areas in terms of the differences in the numbers of practices experiencing a rise in their local populations (Table 4.9). Population rises were significantly higher in the rural/suburban areas (Areas 1, 3 & 4) than in the urban areas (Areas 2, 5, 6 & 7).

Table 4.9
Practices in each area experiencing a population rise

Area	%	no
4. East Rural	55	(22)
3. Thames Valley	44	(14)
1. NW Suburban	37	(15)
6. Midlands Urban	17	(8)
7. North Mining	16	(4)
5. NE Industrial	15	(7)
2. London Inner City	11	(3)
Total	28	(73)

It was also possible to classify the social characteristics of the areas in which individual practices were located (Table 4.10). This table is based on the interviewers' assessment of the area immediately surrounding the practice premises, so should be regarded as a rough indication only.

Area 3 (Thames Valley) had the highest percentage of affluent suburban areas while Area 2 (London Inner City) was largely working class. Area 4 (East Rural) was largely rural while town centre practices were distributed throughout all areas, ranging from 15 per cent of practices in Areas 2 (London Inner City) and 6 (Midlands Urban) to 32 per cent in Areas 1 (NW Suburban) and 5 (NE Industrial).

Practice decisions

1. *Partnership size* Table 4.11 sets out the average number of partners per practice for each study area. The more urban areas (Areas 2, 6, 7) tended to have smaller partnerships than the rural and suburban areas (Areas 1 and 4). The results are presented per full time equivalent partner, with part-timers counted as 0.5.

Table 4.10
Type of location in which the practice was situated

Type of location predominantly:-

Area	Affluent suburban %	no	Working class %	no	Rural %	no	Town centre %	no
3. Thames Valley	69	(22)	13	(4)	0	(0)	19	(6)
1. NW Suburban	34	(14)	17	(7)	17	(7)	32	(13)
6. Midlands Urban	25	(12)	52	(25)	8	(4)	15	(7)
5. NE Industrial	13	(6)	51	(24)	4	(2)	32	(15)
2. London Inner City	4	(1)	82	(22)	0	(0)	15	(4)
4. East Rural	0	(0)	5	(2)	73	(29)	20	(8)
Total	23	(55)	36	(84)	18	(42)	23	(53)

2. *List size* List size varied little with area (Table 4.12). However, the interaction of list size with differences in partnership size between areas (Table 4.11) produced large differences in the average numbers of patients per practice, as shown in Table 4.12. A 16 per cent range in list size was related to a 41 per cent range in the average number of patients per practice. The national policy for equalising list size between areas has had some success, but there were still considerable variations produced by local differences in practice strategy. For the purposes of Table 4.12, list size was per partner, regardless of whether the doctor was full-time or part-time.

Table 4.11
Average partnership size by area

Area	Average no. of partners per practice
1. NW Suburban	3.9
4. East Rural	3.9
5. NE Industrial	3.7
3. Thames Valley	3.5
7. North Mining	3.4
6. Midlands Urban	3.0
2. London Inner City	2.9

Table 4.12
Average list size and average number of patients per practice, by area

Area	Average list size per doctor	Average no. patients per practice
7. North Mining	2258	-
3. Thames Valley	2160	8669
5. NE Industrial	2145	9099
6. Midlands Urban	2106	6753
2. London Inner City	2092	6453
1. NW Suburban	2009	8513
4. East Rural	1940	7899

There were differences between areas in the proportions of practices with an average list size above 2500 (Table 4.13). Area 4 (East Rural) and Area 1 (NW Suburban) had the smallest number of practices with list sizes over 2500, while the highest were in the more urban areas, particularly Area 5 (NE Industrial).

Table 4.13
Practices in each area with average list sizes per doctor of over 2500 and over 2000 patients

	Average list size over 2500		Average list size over 2000	
Area	%	no	%	no
5. NE Industrial	30	(14)	77	(36)
3. Thames Valley	25	(8)	75	(24)
6. Midlands Urban	23	(11)	60	(29)
2. London Inner City	22	(6)	59	(16)
1. NW Suburban	17	(7)	71	(29)
4. East Rural	10	(4)	50	(20)
Total	21	(50)	66	(154)

3. *The employment of practice nurses and other staff* The Family Doctor Charter encouraged the employment of practice nurses. However, there remained a wide variation in the numbers of practices employing a nurse; from 75 per cent of practices in Area 3 (Thames Valley) to 42 per cent in Area 6 (Midlands Urban). There were

special local factors explaining the low proportion of practices employing nurses in Area 7 (North Mining). In this area, District Health Authority nurses were in any case geographically attached, so doctors may not have felt the need to employ their own nurses (Table 4.14). Table 4.15 shows the number of practices in each area employing practice managers. Employment of practice managers was widespread and occurred in 59 per cent of all practices, but was below this proportion in Areas 1, 6 and 7.

Table 4.14
Practices employing at least one nurse
(either full or part-time, SRN or SEN) in each area

Area	%	no
3. Thames Valley	75	(24)
4. East Rural	70	(28)
5. NE Industrial	66	(31)
1. NW Suburban	61	(25)
2. London Inner City	52	(14)
6. Midlands Urban	42	(20)
7. North Mining	28	(7)
Total	57	(149)

Table 4.15
Employment of practice managers (PM)

	% practices with a PM	Part-time PMs		Full-time PMs		Total no. practices
Area		%	no	%	no	
3. Thames Valley	78	38	(12)	41	(13)	32
4. East Rural	73	33	(13)	40	(16)	40
2. London Inner City	70	26	(7)	44	(12)	27
5. NE Industrial	64	15	(7)	49	(23)	47
1. NW Suburban	49	20	(8)	29	(12)	41
6. Midlands Urban	44	19	(9)	25	(12)	48
7. North Mining	40	20	(5)	20	(5)	25
Total	59	24	(61)	36	(93)	260

4. *Participation in the training scheme* The vocational training scheme is usually presented as having been an important step forward for general practice, but the detailed data for the seven areas showed that participation in the scheme was very uneven. The proportions of practices by area which were training practices are set out in Table 4.16. Thus the level of participation varied from 49 per cent of practices in Area 1 (NW Suburban) to only 19 per cent in Areas 5 (NE Industrial) and 6 (Midlands Urban). In all, approximately one third of the responding practices were training practices.

There were 55 practices (23 per cent) in Areas 1-6 which had a trainee at the time of the interview. This figure ranged from 43 per cent of practices in Area 1 (NW Suburban) to only 13 per cent of practices in Area 6 (Midlands Urban).

Table 4.16
Practices in which at least one partner is a trainer

Area	Training practices %	Training practices no	Total no practices
1. NW Suburban	49	(20)	41
4. East Rural	45	(18)	40
2. London Inner City	33	(9)	27
7. North Mining	32	(8)	25
3. Thames Valley	28	(9)	32
5. NE Industrial	19	(9)	47
6. Midlands Urban	19	(9)	48
Total	32	(82)	260

5. *Distribution of dispensing practices* Dispensing practices in each area are listed in Table 4.17. Most were in the rural area (Area 4), though 24 per cent of practices in Area 7 (North Mining) and 17 per cent in Area 1 (NW Suburban) were dispensing practices. There were none in the London Inner City area (Area 2).

6. *Distribution of branch surgeries* Some practices operated from a single location while others had up to four branch surgeries. Branches were often a source of considerable frustration to some doctors because of the difficulty of not knowing which patients would turn up where, with the need either to duplicate notes or risk having to see patients without notes. From Table 4.18 it is clear that branches were more common in the rural area (Area 4), but Area 6 (Midlands Urban) also had a high proportion of practices with at least one branch surgery. The use of branches was lowest in Area 2 (London Inner City), while Area 7 (North Mining) stood out as having by far the highest number of practices with branch premises (84 per cent).

Table 4.17
Distribution of dispensing practices

Area	Dispensing practices %	no	Total no
4. East Rural	68	(27)	40
7. North Mining	24	(6)	25
1. NW Suburban	17	(7)	41
3. Thames Valley	9	(3)	32
5. NE Industrial	4	(2)	47
6. Midlands Urban	4	(2)	48
2. London Inner City	0	(0)	27
Total	18	(47)	260

Table 4.18
Number of practices which have branch surgeries

Area	Practices with at least one branch %	no	Practices with no branches %	no
7. North Mining	84	(21)	16	(4)
4. East Rural	55	(22)	45	(18)
6. Midlands Urban	44	(21)	56	(27)
3. Thames Valley	34	(11)	66	(21)
1. NW Suburban	34	(14)	66	(27)
5. NE Industrial	19	(9)	81	(38)
2. London Inner City	15	(4)	85	(23)
Total	39	(102)	61	(158)

7. *Participation in the cost rent scheme* Another important feature of the Family Doctor Charter was its encouragement to invest in new premises. Here again there was variation in the take-up of the cost rent scheme between areas, the take-up being much higher in the rural area (Area 4) than elsewhere. Here, 75 per cent of the practices had used the scheme, compared with an average for all areas of only 36 per cent. There were also differences in the numbers of practices operating from health centres in each area, and these practices were, by definition, excluded from the cost rent scheme (Table 4.19).

Table 4.19

Participation in the cost rent scheme, and practices in health centres, by area

	Practices using cost rent scheme		Practices in health centres		Total no practices
Area	%	no	%	no	
4. East Rural	75	(30)	20	(8)	40
1. NW Suburban	37	(15)	22	(9)	41
7. North Mining	36	(9)	40	(10)	25
2. London Inner City	33	(9)	33	(9)	27
6. Midlands Urban	27	(13)	31	(15)	48
5. NE Industrial	26	(12)	53	(25)	47
3. Thames Valley	19	(6)	16	(5)	32
Total	36	(94)	31	(81)	260

There were also important differences in the pattern of ownership of practice premises. Table 4.20 sets out the type of ownership of practices in each of the study areas. Collective ownership by the partners predominated (40 per cent), followed by renting from the health authority (30 per cent). Collective ownership predominated in Area 4 (East Rural) (70 per cent), and was fairly evenly distributed in the other 6 areas. Practices were often in health authority premises in Area 5 (NE Industrial) while private renting was most common in Area 1 (NW Suburban) (17 per cent) and Area 3 (Thames Valley) (31 per cent).

8. *Equipment levels* The problems faced by practices investing in working capital have already been mentioned. Again there were substantial differences between areas in the levels of equipment available to practices (Table 4.21). Although over 80 per cent of practices had nebulisers, peak flow meters and proctoscopes, only 25 per cent had haemoglobinometers, although the latter figure varied from 45 per cent in Area 4 (East Rural) to 10 per cent in Area 1 (NW Suburban). Similarly, 60 per cent of all practices had an ECG machine, but this varied from 93 per cent in Area 4 (East Rural) to only 32 per cent in Area 7 (North Mining).

Table 4.20
Ownership of practice premises

Area	Collectively owned %	no	Personally owned %	no	Rented from Health Authority %	no	Privately rented %	no	Other %	no
4. East Rural	70	(28)	8	(3)	20	(8)	3	(1)	0	-
1. NW Suburban	44	(18)	22	(9)	17	(7)	17	(7)	0	-
3. Thames Valley	44	(14)	13	(4)	13	(4)	31	(10)	0	-
5. NE Industrial	38	(18)	4	(2)	53	(25)	4	(2)	0	-
7. North Mining	32	(8)	28	(7)	40	(10)	0	-	0	-
6. Midlands Urban	25	(12)	35	(17)	27	(13)	10	(5)	2	(1)
2. London Inner City	22	(6)	30	(8)	30	(8)	15	(4)	4	(1)
Total	40	(104)	19	(50)	29	(75)	11	(29)	1	(2)

Table 4.21
Percentages of practices owning selected items of equipment in each area

Area	Computer	ECG	Haemoglobinometer	Nebuliser	Proctoscope	Peak flow meter	Total no. practices
4. East Rural	53	93	45	100	88	100	40
3. Thames Valley	50	63	19	88	94	100	32
1. NW Suburban	42	51	10	85	90	98	41
7. North Mining	36	32	36	72	84	96	25
5. NE Industrial	34	83	34	75	81	100	47
6. Midlands Urban	27	42	19	71	79	98	48
2. London Inner City	26	41	15	67	74	100	27
Total	38	60	25	80	84	99	260

There were mixed views of the usefulness of ECG machines to general practices and some conflict was felt with the local hospital. One doctor commented; "It is not necessarily a good idea for doctors to have their own equipment such as ECGs. Doctors don't do enough and can get out of touch with the interpretation of results. It is often better to use the hospital where they are being done all the time". Another sceptical doctor commented in general that he "suspects all the modern aids are just cosmetic".

Although doctors have been encouraged, by various schemes, to invest in computers, only 38 per cent of practices possessed one. The computer was the major item of equipment wanted by doctors who did not have one. Computers were cited 51 times, followed by an ECG machine (41 times), glucometer (19 times), defibrillator (15 times), cautery and audiometer (12 times each).

9. *The provision of off-duty cover* The doctors were asked how their practice covered for partners who were absent or off-duty and the results are set out in Table 4.22. The most popular form of cover was a rota within the partnership, used by 85 per cent of practices. Rota with neighbouring practices was less popular at 24 per cent, but in Area 3 (Thames Valley) this rose to 50 per cent of practices. Locums were used, usually for holiday cover, by 20 per cent of all practices, but by 38 per cent of the Thames Valley practices. The use of deputising services varied according to availability. No service was available to doctors in Area 4 (East Rural) but the service was widely used by 50-60 per cent of the urban practices (Areas 2, 5, 6 and 7).

Table 4.22
How doctors provide cover when off-duty

Area	Rota within partnership %	Deputising services %	Rota with neighbouring practices %	Locum %
7. North Mining	100	68	12	8
4. East Rural	95	0	28	30
6. Midlands Urban	88	52	4	19
2. London Inner City	85	56	7	19
1. NW Suburban	83	7	37	20
5. NE Industrial	77	60	21	11
3. Thames Valley	69	13	50	38
Total	85	35	24	20

Note: Positive responses could be given to more than one alternative.
Figures are percentages of total practices in that area.

Conclusions

The development of the family doctor service has usually been seen in terms of aggregate trends. The aim of this chapter has been to set an alternative focus on local diversity rather than on national trends. The model outlined in Chapter 1 relates general practitioner characteristics, and the local environment to practice decisions on structure. Such a model would only be relevant if there was considerable local variation, and the data from the survey confirm diversity in such indicators as age, sex, ethnic background and membership of professional organisations. The social character and extent of local population increase also vary with the local environment. There are great differences in the decisions made by practices about partnership size, teamwork, participation in the vocational training scheme and in the cost rent scheme. National policy has related to a single entity 'general practice', and the existence of a uniform payment system encourages this approach. This chapter has established the variability of decisions in general practice. The next chapter looks at causation and how different patterns of decision-making by practices relate to differences in personal characteristics and in the local environment.

5 Practice strategies

Chapter 4 presented evidence on local differences in practice decisions. There was considerable local variability which was at odds with the usual picture of changing trends nationally. But in reality, practices do not take decisions in a discrete and unco-ordinated way. Some decisions are more important than others and some are inter-related. This chapter examines decision-making in terms of strategies. A "strategy" involves a co-ordinated series of decisions on the most important issues facing the practice.

In principle, various decisions could be taken as the important ones, and their rankings might change over time, but for the immediate past it is possible to pick out certain decisions which have been the focus for public policy and professional concern. These decisions are the most important for any study of causation of how personal characteristics and local environment affect practice decisions. Improvement of premises, teamwork within the practice through employment of a nurse and participation in the vocational training scheme have been seen as the crucial issues for practice development, attracting both financial support and professional interest. Some doctors may well have been practising excellent medicine in older and unimproved premises, without taking part in the vocational training scheme and without teamwork in the practice: but they were not doing so on the professionally approved model of care (British Medical Association, 1984, Royal College of General Practitioners, 1985).

The hypotheses set out in Chapter 1, could be tested against the evidence in the survey. If the predictions derived from the model were correct, there would firstly be some consistent relationship between personal characteristics and professional motivation in influencing practice decisions; secondly, local environment would be most significant in explaining practice decisions, and thirdly, practices which had been most active in changing their structure and developing services would face the greatest financial pressures.

In order to investigate these factors further, the practices were divided into three groups on the basis of the ways in which they had taken certain decisions.

The factors chosen were, (1) employment of a practice nurse; (2) participation in the cost rent scheme; (3) participation in the vocational training scheme. The employment of a practice nurse was taken as an expression of willingness to incur costs and expand services. Although practices received 70 per cent reimbursement of practice nurse salaries, they nevertheless incurred costs which had to be set against perceived benefits. Practices which had taken part in the cost rent scheme had shown a willingness to invest in their premises and to incur risks. Practices which were training practices had shown a willingness to be subjected to external audit and to maintain certain basic standards. A practice strategy was defined by the choices made on these three issues. These three decisions were not chosen arbitrarily. The development of the vocational training scheme, investment in premises and the development of teamwork have been important aims in policy and have pre-occupied practices locally. Thus a recent report by the Auditor General stressed that "good practice premises help to promote high standards of care and encourage the growth of team work in primary health care. Inadequate accommodation inhibits these developments and limits the range and standard of services provided". (National Audit Office, 1988). The Report also states that "employing ancillary staff helps GPs to provide better and more efficient services for their patients". Practices which took at least two positive decisions were named "innovators"; practices which abstained on all three decisions were known as "traditionalists" and the rest were "intermediates". The survey evidence shows how these three types of practice have distinct strategies and characteristics, not just on the three issues but on a number of others.

For the pilot study, the "low investors" - now designated "traditionalists" - were distinguished using different factors (Bosanquet and Leese, 1986), but the above more unified approach has since been considered more appropriate. As a result, some of the data from the pilot study have been recalculated.

Practices operating from health centres presented particular problems with the classification, since, by their nature, they were unable to take part in the cost rent scheme. This is one reason why "innovators" were designated using two out of three of the chosen characteristics, to allow some health centre practices to fall into this group.

A strategy involves a number of key interdependent decisions which shape a practice's ability to adapt to change and to supply services. Investment in premises is the most long-term decision and conditions the availability of space to the practice. Decisions on staffing critically affect whether partners work as a team, and the range of activities which they undertake. Participation in the training scheme also potentially involves a long-term commitment as well as a willingness to undergo an external audit of the practice. These decisions affect how a practice is seen by fellow professionals, and its impact on patients. There were large differences in the proportions of practices in the various areas which were innovators

(Table 5.1). The proportions of traditionalist practices varied from 44 per cent in Area 7 (North Mining) to 13 per cent in Area 4 (East Rural). Thames Valley (Area 3) might seem to be an apparent exception, as an affluent area without a high proportion of practices which were innovators. However, Thames Valley was made up of two rather different sections. One was much more like an inner city area and among the nine practices in that part of the area there were no innovators. Of 23 practices in the more suburban and affluent section of Thames Valley, 11 or 48 per cent, were innovators. At first sight then, there was a strong association for all areas between practice strategy and the local environment.

Table 5.1
Innovator, intermediate and traditionalist practices by area

	Innovators		Intermediates		Traditionalists	
Area	%	no	%	no	%	no
1. NW Suburban	46	(19)	34	(14)	20	(8)
2. London Inner City	33	(9)	44	(12)	22	(6)
3. Thames Valley	34	(11)	41	(13)	25	(8)
4. East Rural	68	(27)	20	(8)	13	(5)
5. NE Industrial	30	(14)	43	(20)	28	(13)
6. Midlands Urban	23	(11)	38	(18)	40	(19)
7. North Mining	32	(8)	24	(6)	44	(11)
Total	38	(99)	35	(91)	27	(70)

Note: A test of association between area and practice type gave χ^2 calc = 29.13, significant at the 5 per cent level.

Table 5.2 sets out the numbers of individual doctors practising in the three different types of practices. Overall 44 per cent were in innovator practices, compared with only 20 per cent in traditionalist practices, but on an area basis, there were wide differences. For example, the percentages of doctors in innovator practices ranged from 72 per cent of those in Area 4 (East Rural) to only 28 per cent of these in Area 6 (Midlands Urban).

The effect of local environment was examined by classifying the background of the practices across areas (Table 5.3). The classification was made by the interviewer at the time of the interview and was based on the appearance of the area surrounding the practice. This classification does, however, allow for the fact that (for the most part) there are local variations within the relatively large territories covered by FPCs. The evidence also suggests that there are effects from local environment. Forty per cent of practices in an affluent and suburban environment were innovators and only

16 per cent were traditionalists. 57 per cent of practices in rural areas were innovators and 17 per cent traditionalists. In other areas, innovators amounted to about one third of practices and the traditionalists to another third.

Table 5.2
Doctors in each type of practice, by area

Area	Innovators %	no	Intermediates %	no	Traditionalists %	no	Total no
4. East Rural	72	(114)	17	(27)	11	(18	159
1. NW Suburban	51	(87)	32	(55)	17	(30)	172
2. London Inner City	46	(38)	40	(33)	15	(12)	83
3. Thames Valley	39	(49)	47	(59)	15	(19)	127
7. North Mining	38	(33)	25	(22)	37	(32)	87
5. NE Industrial	35	(67)	46	(89)	19	(37)	193
6. Midlands Urban	28	(41)	39	(58)	34	(50)	149
Total	44	(429)	35	(343)	20	(198)	970

Table 5.3
Local environment and practice type

Area	Innovators %	no	Intermediates %	no	Traditionalists %	no	Total
1. Rural	57	(24)	26	(11)	17	(7)	42
2. Affluent Suburban	40	(22)	44	(24)	16	(9)	55
3. Urban	34	(18)	34	(18)	32	(17)	53
4. Working Class	31	(26)	38	(32)	31	(26)	84

[Area 7 North Mining excluded]

Note: A test of association between local environment and practice type gave χ^2 calc = 12.5; significant at the 5 per cent level.

There was one other feature of the local environment which was associated with innovation. This was the degree of change in the local population. Innovating practices were much more likely to have experienced a rise in the local population surrounding the practices (Table 5.4). The association was clearest in the NW Suburban, Thames Valley, East Rural and Midlands Urban areas. In these areas from 46 to 73 per cent of the innovators had experienced an increase in the local population around the practice.

Table 5.4
Practices experiencing a population rise in their area

	Innovators		Intermediates		Traditionalists		Total	
Area	%	no	%	no	%	no	%	no
3. Thames Valley	73	(8)	31	(4)	25	(2)	44	(14)
1. NW Suburban	58	(11)	14	(2)	25	(2)	37	(15)
4. East Rural	56	(15)	63	(5)	40	(2)	55	(22)
6. Midlands Urban	46	(5)	11	(2)	5	(1)	17	(8)
7. North Mining	25	(2)	0	(0)	18	(2)	16	(4)
5. NE Industrial	14	(2)	15	(3)	15	(2)	15	(7)
2. London Inner City	11	(1)	17	(2)	0	(0)	11	(3)
Total	44	(44)	20	(18)	16	(11)	28	(73)

The decision to innovate will now be considered in more detail. Table 5.5 sets out the proportions of innovator practices taking each of the three chosen decisions on practice strategy and compares them with "intermediates". Traditionalists had by definition not taken any of these decisions, so are excluded from this Table.

Participation in the training scheme was the clearest distinguishing feature followed by use of the cost rent scheme. Six out of ten of the intermediate practices were employing a nurse. In general the innovators were very likely to have taken all three decisions. 73 per cent were training practices, 72 per cent were taking part in the cost rent scheme and 92 per cent were employing a nurse.

How did the choices made by practices affect the numbers of patients registered with different types of practice? Overall, 44 per cent of patients were registered with innovator practices, but this proportion varied from 71 per cent in the East Rural area to 27 per cent in the Midlands Urban area (Table 5.6).

Table 5.5
Training practices, practices employing a nurse and practices which have taken part in the cost rent scheme by area and practice type

Area	Training: Innovators %	Training: Intermediates %	Nurses: Innovators %	Nurses: Intermediates %	Cost rent: Innovators %	Cost rent: Intermediates %
1. NW Suburban	89*	21	84	64	68	14
2. London Inner City	78	17	100	42	56	33
3. Thames Valley	82	0	100	100	55	0
4. East Rural	63	13	93	38	93	63
5. NE Industrial	64	0	100	85	64	15
6. Midlands Urban	64	11	100	50	55	39
7. North Mining	75	33	63	33	88	33
Total	73	11	92	64	72	25

* Figures are % of practices in that area and practice type which are training practices, etc.

Table 5.6
Percentages of patients in each practice type, by area

Area	Innovators %	Intermediates %	Traditionalists %	Total number of patients (000)
1. NW Suburban	51	30	19	316.0
2. London Inner City	46	40	14	174.2
3. Thames Valley	40	45	15	277.4
4. East Rural	71	18	11	316.0
5. NE Industrial	34	47	19	418.5
6. Midlands Urban	27	40	33	323.2
Total	44	37	19	1825.3

Practice strategy: causation

It will be recalled that the aim of this chapter was to examine the relationship between certain key variables and practice decisions. The key variables are to do with a range of personal characteristics and with the impact of the local environment. At first sight there might seem to be a strong and clear relationship between practice strategy and the local environment, but a more detailed analysis is required as to whether the area effect simply masks differences in personal characteristics. For example there could be differences in age structure among general practitioners so that areas with higher proportions of younger doctors might see more innovation. Environmentally attractive areas might recruit doctors with distinctive professional backgrounds. The area effect might also be a proxy for differences between practices of different sizes. Larger practices might be more likely to innovate whatever area they were in. These are still area effects, but they must be more precisely defined.

1. *Age* There was some relationship between innovation and the average age of the partners. Partnerships with a younger average age were more likely to be innovators. The effect was particularly strong in Area 2 (London Inner City) where the average age of partners in traditionalist practices was 52.8 years and for innovators 41.5 years (Table 5.7).

Table 5.7
Average age of partners, by area (years)

Area	Innovators	Intermediates	Traditionalists
1. NW Suburban	42.8	43.5	44.6
2. London Inner City	41.5	46.4	52.8
3. Thames Valley	41.9	46.3	42.9
4. East Rural	43.5	39.9	46.3
5. NE Industrial	40.0	42.8	43.5
6. Midlands Urban	42.8	45.8	44.9
7.North Mining	39.5	49.3	45.9

Overall, differences in the age distribution of doctors between areas were small. If younger doctors were much more likely to be in innovatory practices, an area with a higher proportion of younger doctors would be expected to have more innovatory practices. There was some effect of this kind in areas where the proportion of older doctors was very high. Two of the areas (London Inner City and Midlands Urban) with the lowest proportion of innovator practices also had the highest proportions of practices where the average age of partners was over 50 years, but in general, differences were greater than could be explained by differences in the age distribution of doctors.

2. *Sex* The presence of a female partner in a practice had some relationship to practice strategy. 55 per cent of innovator practices had female partners compared to 37 per cent of traditionalist practices (Table 5.8). In this respect there were significant differences between innovators and traditionalists both in areas with large numbers of female doctors and in areas such as North Mining where there were many fewer female doctors.

Table 5.8
Practices with at least one female partner

	Innovators		Intermediates		Traditionalists	
Area	%	no	%	no	%	no
1. NW Suburban	79	(15)	50	(7)	62	(5)
2. London Inner City	89	(8)	83	(10)	17	(1)
3. Thames Valley	45	(5)	77	(10)	50	(4)
4. East Rural	33	(9)	25	(2)	20	(1)
5. NE Industrial	50	(7)	60	(12)	39	(5)
6. Midlands Urban	45	(5)	44	(8)	42	(8)
7. North Mining	63	(5)	33	(2)	9	(1)
Total	55	(54)	56	(51)	36	(25)

3. *Ethnic background* The ethnic background of the partners was related to differences in practice strategy. Doctors of Asian origin were more likely than other doctors to be in traditionalist practices. Over all areas, 28 per cent of doctors in traditionalist practices were Asian, compared with only 9 per cent and 8 per cent of all doctors in innovator and intermediate practices respectively.

However, the situation is more complex, as illustrated in Table 5.9, which sets out the number of practices in each area and practice type which have at least one Asian partner. Here, 47 per cent of traditionalist practices had at least one Asian partner as did 30 per cent of innovator practices, but only 13 per cent of intermediates. All except three areas had a higher proportion of Asians in traditionalist practices. The exceptions were Area 5 (NE Industrial) and Area 6 (Midlands Urban) where a higher percentage of innovator practices had at least one Asian partner and Area 4 (East Rural) where the only Asian doctor was in an intermediate practice. These results suggested that the Asian doctors in innovator practices were spread more thinly than were the Asian doctors in intermediate and traditional practices. There were 38 Asian doctors in 30 innovator practices (a mean of 1.37 per practice), 27 Asian doctors in 12 intermediate practices (a mean of 2.35 per practice) and 56 Asian doctors in 33 traditionalist practices (a mean of 1.7 per practice).

Table 5.9
Number of practices in each area and practice type with at least one Asian partner

Area	All %	All no	Innovators %	Innovators no	Intermediates %	Intermediates no	Traditionalists %	Traditionalists no
7. North Mining	60	(15)	50	(4)	50	(3)	73	(8)
6. Midlands Urban	42	(20)	73	(8)	22	(4)	42	(8)
5. NE Industrial	40	(19)	64	(9)	10	(2)	62	(8)
2. London Inner City	37	(10)	44	(4)	17	(2)	67	(4)
3. Thames Valley	16	(5)	18	(2)	0	(0)	38	(3)
1. NW Suburban	12	(5)	16	(3)	0	(0)	25	(2)
4. East Rural	3	(1)	0	(0)	13	(1)	0	(0)
Total	29	(75)	30	(30)	13	(12)	47	(33)

4. *Length of service* There were some (but small) differences in length of service. The average length of service by partners in their present practice was 12 years for innovators compared with 13 years for intermediates. The traditionalist average length of service was particularly high in the North East Industrial area (17 years) and in the Midlands Urban area (15 years). But in general the range of variation was too small to show much effect on decisions about strategy.

5. *The nature of the contract* There were also few differences in the proportions of part-time family doctors between practices with different strategies. 33 per cent of innovators had at least one part-time partner compared with 35 per cent of intermediates and 38 per cent of traditionalists. The balance was however rather different from the point of view of the doctor seeking part-time employment. As there were many more innovator and intermediate practices they were able to recruit more part-time staff. Of the 95 part-time partners in the survey, 41 were in innovator practices, 40 in intermediate and only 14 in traditionalist practices.

6. *Membership of professional organisations* There were only small differences in membership of the BMA between practice types (Table 5.10). However 42 per cent of innovator practices had at least one partner who was a member of the RCGP compared to only 22 per cent of traditionalist practices, and RCGP membership was particularly high among innovator practices in three of the four less affluent areas (Areas 2, 5 and 7).

Table 5.10
Membership of professional organisations by area and practice type

Area	Membership of BMA Innovators %	Intermediates %	Traditionalists %	Membership of RCGP Innovators %	Intermediates %	Traditionalists %
1. NW Suburban	75	44	47	38	22	23
2. London Inner City	92	91	50	47	33	33
3. Thames Valley	69	68	74	51	19	37
4. East Rural	68	56	50	31	22	11
5. NE Industrial	87	71	78	63	40	22
6. Midlands Urban	73	81	70	29	31	20
7. North Mining	67	45	31	39	5	6
Total	76	69	64	42	29	22

7. *Outside posts* Doctors from innovator practices were somewhat more likely to have posts outside general practice. Overall 82 per cent of innovator practices had partners with outside posts compared to 75 per cent of traditionalist practices (Table 5.11).

Table 5.11
Practices in which at least one partner had outside post(s)

Area	Innovators %	no	Intermediates %	no	Traditionalists %	no	Total %	no
1. NW Suburban	100	(19)	86	(12)	50	(4)	85	(35)
2. London Inner City	100	(9)	67	(8)	67	(4)	78	(21)
3. Thames Valley	100	(11)	85	(11)	75	(6)	88	(28)
5. NE Industrial	79	(11)	95	(19)	69	(9)	83	(39)
4. East Rural	74	(20)	38	(3)	60	(3)	65	(26)
6. Midlands Urban	36	(4)	72	(13)	95	(18)	73	(35)
Total	82	(74)	78	(66)	75	(44)	78	(184)

Other elements in strategy

1. *Practice managers* Innovator practices also differed in other decisions which they made. They were more likely to employ practice managers (Table 5.12).

Table 5.12
Practices having at least one full-time or part-time practice manager

	Innovators		Intermediates		Traditionalists		Total	
Area	%	no	%	no	%	no	%	no
3. Thames Valley	*91	(10)	77	(10)	63	(5)	78	(25)
2. London Inner City	89	(8)	75	(9)	33	(2)	70	(19)
5. NE Industrial	86	(12)	65	(13)	39	(5)	64	(30)
4. East Rural	82	(22)	50	(4)	60	(3)	73	(29)
7. North Mining	75	(6)	50	(3)	9	(1)	40	(10)
1. NW Suburban	74	(14)	36	(5)	13	(1)	49	(20)
6. Midlands Urban	64	(7)	33	(6)	42	(8)	44	(21)
Total	80	(79)	55	(50)	36	(25)	59	(154)

* % of stated practice type in each area which have practice managers.

2. *Equipment* The possession of specific items of equipment differed depending on the type of practice. Innovator practices were much more likely to have computers. 59 per cent of innovator practices had a computer compared with 34 per cent of intermediates and only 14 per cent of traditionalists (Table 5.13). There were similar differences when other items of equipment were considered. For example, ECG machines were owned by 77 per cent of innovator practices, 57 per cent of intermediates and only 40 per cent of traditionalists.

3. *Partnership size* The trend to larger practices has always been seen as significant. How far are the variations in practice size dependent on practice strategy? In order to answer this question, partnership size was measured in terms of the average number of partners per practice.

There were differences in average numbers of partners between types of practice. Overall, traditionalist practices averaged 2.7 partners, intermediates 3.4 and innovator practices 4.1 (Table 5.14). Area 2 (London Inner City) had the lowest average partnership size, of 2.9. The highest average partnership size of 3.9 was found in both the NW Suburban and the East Rural area even though as an area of scattered population, this must have meant considerable travelling difficulties for some patients in the latter area.

Table 5.13
Practices having the listed items of equipment

Equipment	Innovators n=99 %	Innovators no	Intermediates n=91 %	Intermediates no	Traditionalists n=70 %	Traditionalists no	Total %	Total no
Computer	59	(58)	34	(31)	14	(10)	38	(99)
ECG	77	(76)	57	(52)	40	(28)	60	(156)
Haemoglobinometer	30	(30)	25	(23)	19	(13)	25	(66)
Nebuliser	95	(94)	75	(69)	61	(43)	79	(206)
Peak flow meter	100	(99)	100	(91)	96	(67)	99	(257)
Proctoscope	87	(86)	84	(76)	81	(57)	84	(219)

Table 5.14
Average number of partners per practice

Area	All types	Innovators	Intermediates	Traditionalists
1. NW Suburban	3.9	4.3	3.5	3.6
2. London Inner City	2.9	4.0	2.5	1.9
3. Thames Valley	3.5	4.2	3.8	2.3
4. East Rural	3.9	4.1	3.3	3.4
5. NE Industrial	3.7	4.4	3.8	2.7
6. Midlands Urban	3.0	3.6	3.2	2.6
Total	3.5	4.1	3.4	2.7

Note: Part-time partners counted as 0.5. Data are therefore based on full-time equivalent partners.

It was also possible to see how partnership size had changed over the ten years 1976-1986 (Table 5.15). Innovator practices were larger to start with and had grown since, so that by 1986, average partnership size was greater than four in all but one area. Traditionalist practices had shown most growth in more affluent areas such as NW Suburban and East Rural. It was also in those areas that traditionalist practices had been most likely to experience a rise in their local population.

Table 5.15
Average number of partners per practice over ten years

Area	10 years ago (1976)	Now (1986)	% change 1976-1986
1. NW Suburban			
Innovator	3.5	4.6	+31
Intermediate	3.1	3.8	+23
Traditionalist	2.6	3.7	+42
All	3.2	4.1	+28
2. London Inner City			
Innovator	3.2	4.2	+31
Intermediate	2.1	2.7	+29
Traditionalist	1.5	2.0	+33
All	2.3	3.1	+35
3. Thames Valley			
Innovator	3.6	4.4	+22
Intermediate	3.9	4.1	+5
Traditionalist	2.0	2.4	+20
All	3.3	3.8	+15
4. East Rural			
Innovator	3.4	4.2	+23
Intermediate	3.4	3.4	0
Traditionalist	2.4	3.6	+50
All	3.2	4.0	+25
5. NE Industrial			
Innovator	4.1	4.8	+17
Intermediate	3.8	4.2	+11
Traditionalist	2.1	3.0	+43
All	3.4	4.0	+18
6. Midlands Urban			
Innovator	2.1	3.7	+76
Intermediate	2.9	3.2	+10
Traditionalist	2.5	2.5	0
All	2.5	3.0	+20
7. North Mining			
Innovator	3.6	4.1	+14
Intermediate	3.2	3.6	+12
Traditionalist	3.3	3.0	-9
All	3.4	3.4	0

The relationship between partnership size and strategy was also examined more directly. As Table 5.16 shows, there was a strong relationship between innovation and size of practice. Practices with four partners or more were much more likely to have become innovators than smaller ones. Thus, 19 per cent of two partner practices were innovators compared with 72 per cent of five partner practices.

Table 5.16
Strategy and size of practice

Number of partners	Innovators %	Innovators no	Intermediates %	Intermediates no	Traditionalists %	Traditionalists no	Total number of practices
2	19	(12)	30	(19)	52	(33)	64
3	27	(21)	42	(32)	31	(24)	77
4	44	(22)	38	(19)	18	(9)	50
5	72	(21)	24	(7)	3	(1)	29
6	64	(16)	28	(7)	8	(2)	25
7	50	(5)	40	(4)	10	(1)	10
8	0	(0)	100	(1)	0	(0)	1
9	100	(2)	0	(0)	0	(0)	2
10	0	(0)	100	(2)	0	(0)	2

The relationship between innovation and practice size was a little more complex at the area level. In the more affluent areas, (NW Suburban, East Rural), smaller practices were more likely to innovate. The majority of larger practices were innovators in all areas, but there seems to be an area effect on smaller practices (Table 5.17).

Practices in the London Inner City area faced particular problems in the form of high property prices and difficulties in finding sites for cost-rented premises, which may have been factors in keeping partnership size lower.

Table 5.17
Innovation and smaller practices by area

Number of partners	Innovators: NW Suburban %*	NW Suburban no	London Inner City %	London Inner City no	Thames Valley %	Thames Valley no	East Rural %	East Rural no	NE Industrial %	NE Industrial no	Midlands Urban %	Midlands Urban no
2	43	(3)	9	(3)	11	(1)	29	(2)	14	(1)	13	(2)
3	14	(1)	36	(4)	43	(3)	69	(9)	7	(1)	10	(2)

*percentage of practices of a given size within the area

Table 5.18
Changes in list size per partner*

Area	Ten years ago	Now	% Change
1. NW Suburban			
Innovator	2274	2021	-11
Intermediate	2182	1899	-13
Traditionalist	2570	2170	-16
All	2287	2009	-12
2. London Inner City			
Innovator	2432	2113	-13
Intermediate	2072	2076	-
Traditional	2230	2092	-6
All	2219	2092	-6
3. Thames Valley			
Innovator	2138	2232	+4
Intermediate	2260	2058	-9
Traditionalist	2105	2226	+6
All	2179	2160	-1
4. East Rural			
Innovator	2062	1899	-8
Intermediate	2061	2136	+4
Traditionalist	2517	1852	-26
All	2111	1940	-8
5. NE Industrial			
Innovator	2460	2124	-14
Intermediate	2507	2192	-13
Traditionalist	3003	2102	-30
All	2628	2145	-18
6. Midlands Urban			
Innovator	2254	2021	-10
Intermediate	2436	2163	-11
Traditionalist	2245	2101	-6
All	2320	2106	-9
7. North Mining			
Innovator	2465	2123	-14
Intermediate	2670	2411	-10
Traditionalist	2700	2206	-18
All	2610	2258	-14

* Total numbers of partners unweighted for part-timers

4. *List size* List size has been an important variable in terms of national policy and considerable effort has been expended on reducing average list size between FPC areas across the country. This effort has been largely successful.

List size has fallen in all areas and the equalisation encouraged by policy incentives has taken place (Butler, Bevan and Taylor, 1973). Innovator practices had list sizes ten years ago that were below the area average in six of the areas. Their list sizes continued to fall, but the largest changes were found among traditionalist practices. In four areas - NW Suburban, East Rural, NE Industrial and N Mining - list sizes in traditionalist practices fell by much more than the area average (Table 5.18).

List size now shows little variation between area and type of practice. Thus it does not in itself appear to be a significant variable affecting practice strategy, but differences in partnership size interact with what differences there are in list size to produce large differences in total numbers of patients between practice types (Table 5.19).

Thus, differences in practice strategy may not affect list size for each partner, but they do influence total practice size and the number of patients which a practice serves.

Table 5.19
Average number of patients and average list size by practice type

Practice type	Number of patients	Average list size
Innovators	9033	2035
Intermediates	8101	2094
Traditionalists	6033	2105
All	7942	2074

Statistical analysis of practice strategy

A more formal statistical analysis of the relationships between personal characteristics, local environment and strategy was carried out. The full results are set out in Appendix 1. The study used the technique of logit modelling which is more suitable for data of this kind than conventional regression analysis. The key decision to be explored was the decision to innovate. This was done in relation to the practices which were innovators or traditionalists. A number of key variables were assessed in relation to the decision to innovate. These included:

Average age of the partnership.
Practices with and without female partners.
Ethnic background.
Membership of professional organisations.
Area in which the practice was situated.
Partnership size.

The main results were as follows:

(1) The average age of the partnership was a significant factor in affecting innovation. More elderly partnerships were less likely to be innovative.

(2) The sex of the partners has no effect on innovation. The presence or absence of a female doctor did not affect innovation one way or the other.

(3) The ethnic background of the partners was significant in affecting innovation. Practices with Asian partners were less likely to innovate.

(4) Membership by one or more partners in the Royal College of General Practitioners was significantly associated with innovation, especially in the less affluent areas.

(5) The area in which the practice was situated had a significant effect on innovation. In particular, practices in the East Rural area were more likely to innovate.

(6) Partnership size was significantly associated with innovation. Partnership size and area were significantly inter-related so that either variable was significant independently, but not both together.

Thus, age, ethnic background, area and partnership size were all significant variables in affecting the decision to innovate. The full results together with appropriate tests are set out in Appendix 1.

Conclusions

In this chapter, the main patterns of causation have been examined. Area has been found to be a complex variable, where such factors as size of practice and different ethnic backgrounds turn out to be important. In general the first two hypotheses tested received support in that there was a systematic relationship on an area basis between practice decisions and external variables. Practices in more affluent areas with expanding populations were more likely to innovate, but area was found to be a term which covered a complex set of interactions.

In the following chapters, detailed data on outcomes and patient services are presented.

6 Outcomes for doctors

This chapter looks at the ways in which the different practice strategies described in Chapter 5 affect the "outcomes" for the doctors themselves in terms of their incomes, practice costs and capital investment. Within the model (Figure 1.1), personal characteristics, the payment system and the local environment, condition decisions on practice structure and strategy which then lead to outcomes in terms of economic consequences for the practices. This chapter begins by summarising the evidence on outcomes collected from the survey. This is treated in some detail as it represents the first available data on the incomes of family doctors on a small area basis. Data were collected on the following main variables:

Gross income: This was defined as total income from Family Practitioner Committee sources in fees and allowances, excluding direct re-imbursement of rent, rates, and ancillary staff salaries.
Net income: This was the amount of income available for distribution among the partners after paying all costs, but before the payment of personal taxation i.e. the practice 'profits'.
Practice costs: The difference between 'gross' and 'net' income as defined above.
Capital value: The estimated market value of the practice premises, where applicable.

Efforts were made to ensure the accuracy of the income data. Wherever possible, figures were taken from the most recent practice accounts. Figures collected by interviewers were checked in follow up telephone calls with practices as necessary.

Reluctant responders were asked to indicate the practice income from a set of possible ranges offered. The average figures for gross and net income collected in the survey correspond closely with the data collected in the Review Body Report for 1986/7 (Review Body on Doctors and Dentists Remuneration, 1987).

The results in Chapter 5 suggested that there were strong area effects on practice strategy, but that 'area' was a complex variable reflecting differences in partnership size, age structure, and the ethnic background of the partners.

In this chapter, the relationships between practice strategy and financial outcomes are explored with reference to area, innovation and income.

Income and area

There was considerable variation in income between areas, as can be seen in Table 6.1. The variations in average net income between areas were larger than those in average gross income. Excluding the East Rural area with its special effects from the presence of dispensing income, levels of average gross income between areas were similar, NW Suburban (£40,900), Thames Valley (£39,800), North East Industrial (£38,900) and Midlands Urban (£37,000). Differences in costs between areas lead to greater differences in average net income than were seen for average gross income.

Table 6.1
Gross and net incomes and costs (£,000)

Area	Mean gross income per partner	Mean net income per partner	Cost ratios: net to gross income	Co-efficient of variation of gross income	Co-efficient of variation of net income
1. NW Suburban	40.9	26.3	.64	36.3	20.5
3. Thames Valley	39.8	29.2	.73	31.9	23.1
4. East Rural*	72.0	33.7	.47	42.5	23.1
2. London Inner City	33.6	23.3	.69	28.6	26.6
5. North East Industrial	38.9	27.1	.70	21.8	23.1
6. Midlands Urban	37.0	23.9	.65	32.7	29.2
All	43.8	27.3	.62	-	-
7. North Mining**	32.2	22.7	.70	-	-

* Includes gross costs associated with dispensing.
** Data collected one year earlier than in other areas.

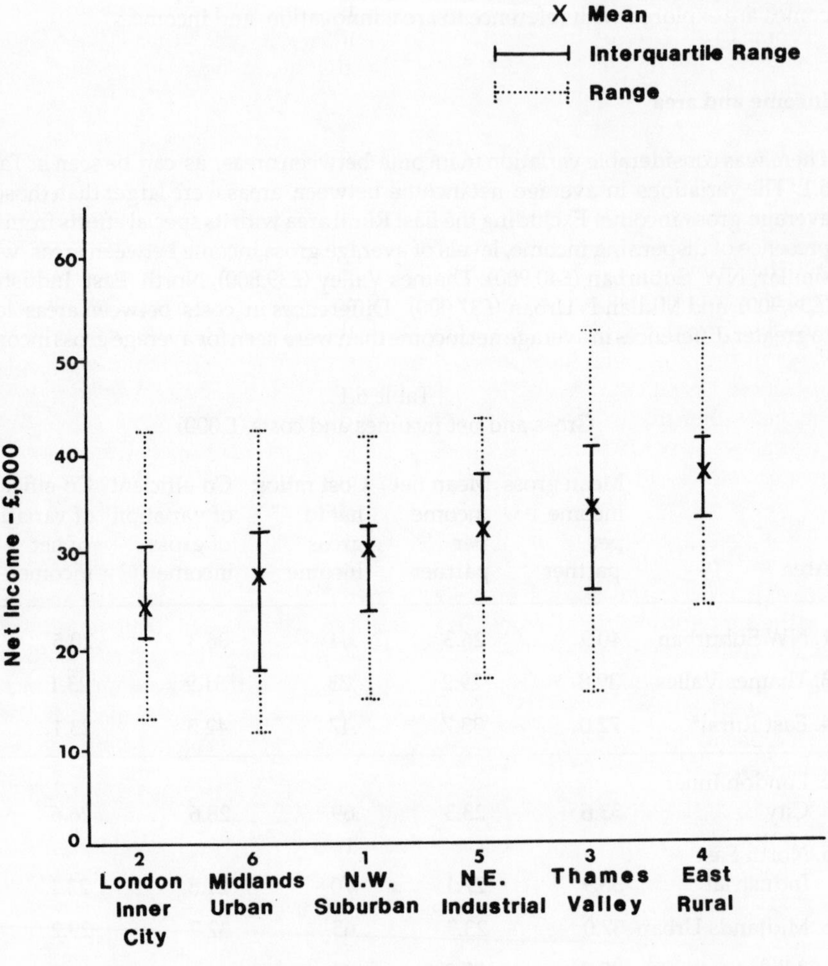

Figure 6.1 Net income per partner, by area

There were also some differences in the variability of income within areas. The coefficient of variation of gross income by area is generally higher than for net income, apart from Area 5 (North East Industrial) where a higher proportion of practices were in health centres. There are clearly major variations between practices, within areas, in their ability to control costs. For net income, the coefficient of variation was highest in two of the urban areas, (Midlands Urban and London Inner City). Thus in the Midlands Urban area the coefficient of variation was 29 per cent and in the London Inner City area it was 27 per cent, compared to 20-23 per cent in the other areas. These variations are illustrated in Figure 6.1. The bottom quartile was at a lower level of income in the London Inner City and Midlands Urban areas. The widest range was to be found in the Thames Valley area reflecting the unusual mix of inner city and affluent suburbs to be found there.

Income and practice strategy

Table 6.2 sets out income levels in practices with different strategies.

The average levels of net income achieved by innovators were more diverse than those of traditionalists. In affluent areas, innovators had net incomes which were much higher than the average for all areas in the survey. Thus, in the Thames Valley area the income of innovator practices was 23 per cent above the average for all practices in the survey, and in the East Rural area it was 27 per cent above, while in the London Inner City area the net incomes of innovators were 6 per cent below the average of all practices in the survey (see Table 6.2). The traditionalists' income was comparatively low and did not show any marked differences between areas.

In general, although the average incomes of the innovators were higher, this was not a good indication of the returns to be expected from innovation in the less affluent areas. The innovators in the NW Suburban, Thames Valley, and East Rural areas had net incomes which were well above the averages achieved by all practices in the study or in their areas, but this was not so in other areas. In the London Inner City, Midlands Urban and North Mining areas, innovators had higher costs than the average for their areas and this was a major factor in determining net income.

A stepwise regression analysis was carried out to identify the effects of list size, area, partnership size and practice strategy on income. The main results can be summarised as follows:

a) List size had an important effect on practice net income.
b)Practices in three areas; London Inner City (Area 2), Thames Valley (Area 3) and East Rural (Area 4) had net incomes which were significantly different from those in other areas.
c) Partnership size was significant in affecting net income if the list size variable was excluded.
d) Practice strategy had some effect on income. Practices which did not innovate had lower net incomes.

Other variables such as the presence or absence of Asian or female partners did not have an influence on average net incomes.

Table 6.2
Average gross and net income per (full-time equivalent) partner by area and practice type 1986-7

	Gross income per partner (£,000)	Net income per partner (£,000)	Cost ratio: net to gross income
1. NW Suburban			
Innovator	42.9	27.8	.65
Intermediate	39.4	26.2	.66
Traditionalist	38.0	22.4	.59
All	41.0	26.3	.64
3. Thames Valley			
Innovator	44.8	33.6	.75
Intermediate	39.0	29.3	.75
Traditionalist	34.7	22.8	.66
All	39.8	29.2	.73
4. East Rural			
Innovator	75.6	34.6	.46
Intermediate	73.0	33.4	.46
Traditionalist	48.5	28.5	.59
All	72.0	33.7	.47
2. London Inner City			
Innovator	38.3	25.7	.67
Intermediate	31.6	21.9	.69
Traditionalist	30.6	22.3	.73
All	33.6	23.3	.69
5. NE Industrial			
Innovator	38.0	27.5	.72
Intermediate	40.6	28.5	.70
Traditionalist	38.1	25.3	.66
All	38.9	27.1	.70
6. Midlands Urban			
Innovator	40.4	25.0	.62
Intermediate	37.1	23.8	.64
Traditionalist	34.8	23.3	.67
All	37.0	23.9	.65
All			
Innovator	50.4	29.7	.59
Intermediate	43.2	26.9	.62
Traditionalist	36.7	24.0	.65
All	43.8	27.3	.62
7. North Mining			
Innovator	36.3	23.4	.64
Intermediate	36.7	26.3	.72
Traditionalist	27.1	20.7	.76
All	32.2	22.7	.70

In summary, the best explanatory equation of net income contained the following independent variables:

Patients per full time equivalent doctor	$\beta = 0.509541$
Practices in East Rural/not in East Rural	$\beta = 0.445954$
Innovator or not	$\beta = -0.198726$
Practices in London Inner City/ not in London Inner City	$\beta = -0.115237$
Practices in Thames Valley/ not in Thames Valley	$\beta = 0.107342$

Multiple correlation = 0.67367 (R^2 = 0.45396)
All independent variables significant at the 5 per cent level.

Income and partnership size

The importance of partnership size is further illustrated in Table 6.3 and in Figure 6.2.

Table 6.3
Net and gross income per partner and costs, by partnership size (£,000)

Number of partners	Average net income	Average gross income	Cost ratio: net to gross income	Number of practices
2	21.8	40.3	.54	52
3	25.5	41.9	.61	63
4	27.6	43.8	.63	39
5	27.7	41.2	.67	23
6	30.3	45.0	.67	21
7+	26.4	34.8	.76	12
Mean	25.8	41.5	.62	210

Practices with 3 or fewer partners had lower average net incomes and higher costs than other practices. The optimum scale of operation appeared to be in partnerships with 5 or 6 partners, which had lower costs and higher net incomes. Practices with 7 or more partners had low costs but also low gross and net incomes. The trend towards a middle partnership size range, which has been encouraged by policy, also has a financial logic.

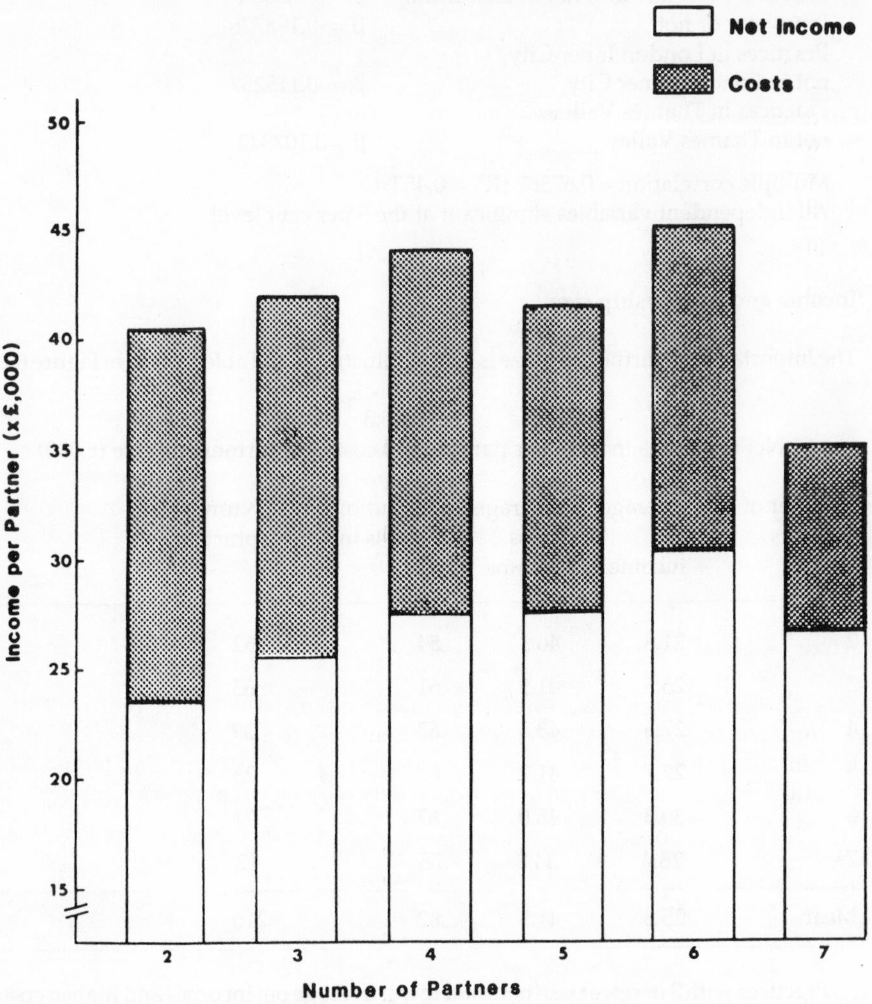

Figure 6.2. Net income and costs per partner by partnership size (the total column height represents gross income)

Income and age

Table 6.4 sets out the results showing the effect of age on incomes.

Table 6.4
Variations with age in net income per partner

Average age of partners in the practice(years)	Average net income (£,000)	Numbers of practices
30 - 39.9	26.2	61
40 - 49.9	28.5	127
50 - 59.9	23.4	22
60+	25.3	5
Total	25.9	215

Practices in which the average age of the partners was over 50 years had lower average net incomes than practices with a younger average age, but numbers with this higher average age were small (13 per cent of responding practices). In general, the effect of the partnership system is to reduce the impact of age on earnings, because partners share income and costs equally once they have reached parity.

Income and health centres

Table 6.5 shows the effect on incomes of practising from a health centre. Costs were found to be lower on average in health centres, but net incomes were similar. These findings may help to explain the low level of costs in the North East Industrial area (Table 6.1) where there were large numbers of practices in health centres.

Table 6.5
Incomes and health centres (£,000)

	In a health centre		Not in a health centre	
Income	£	no	£	no
Average gross income per partner	40.8	(66)	45.1	(151)
Average net income per partner	27.1	(65)	27.3	(150)
Average gross income per practice	136.8	(66)	161.2	(151)
Average net income per practice	93.4	(65)	102.8	(150)
Net:gross ratio per partner	0.66		0.61	

Low and high incomes

The data were also analysed to assess the variability in practice incomes across all areas. The data are presented in Table 6.6 and in graphical form in Figure 6.3.

Table 6.6
Practices having specified net incomes per (full time equivalent) partner

Income range	no	%	cumulative %
0-15000	17	7.9	7.9
15001-20000	28	13.0	20.9
20001-25000	50	23.3	44.2
25001-30000	58	27.0	71.2
30001-35000	31	14.4	85.6
35001-40000	17	7.9	93.5
40001-45000	8	3.7	97.2
45001-50000	6	2.8	100.0
Total	215	100.0	100.0

21 per cent of practices had average net incomes per doctor of £20,000 a year or less and a further 29 per cent had average net incomes per partner above £30,000 a year.

An analysis was carried out of partnerships with 'low' and 'high' incomes. There were 45 practices in the six areas of the main study, or 21 per cent of the total, which had a net income per (full time equivalent) partner of £20,000 or under. Of these 45 practices, nine had partners with an average age above fifty, and 21 had at least one Asian partner. Thus there were a number of practices with both low incomes and Asian partners. These practices were mainly found in urban areas. Of the 45 low income practices, 16 (36 per cent) were in the Midlands Urban area and eight (18 per cent) in the London Inner City area.

An analysis of practices with high incomes, defined as those with a net income per (full time equivalent) partner above £30,000, showed that there were 62 such practices, or 29 per cent of practices in the survey. The chances of high income varied by size of practice and area (Tables 6.7 and 6.8).

High income practices were most common among practices with 5-7 partners and in the East Rural and Thames Valley areas.

The frequency of high and low incomes was also related to practice strategy. Table 6.9 sets out the proportions of practices in the main income bands. Thus, 39 per cent of traditionalist practices had low incomes while 42 per cent of innovators had high incomes.

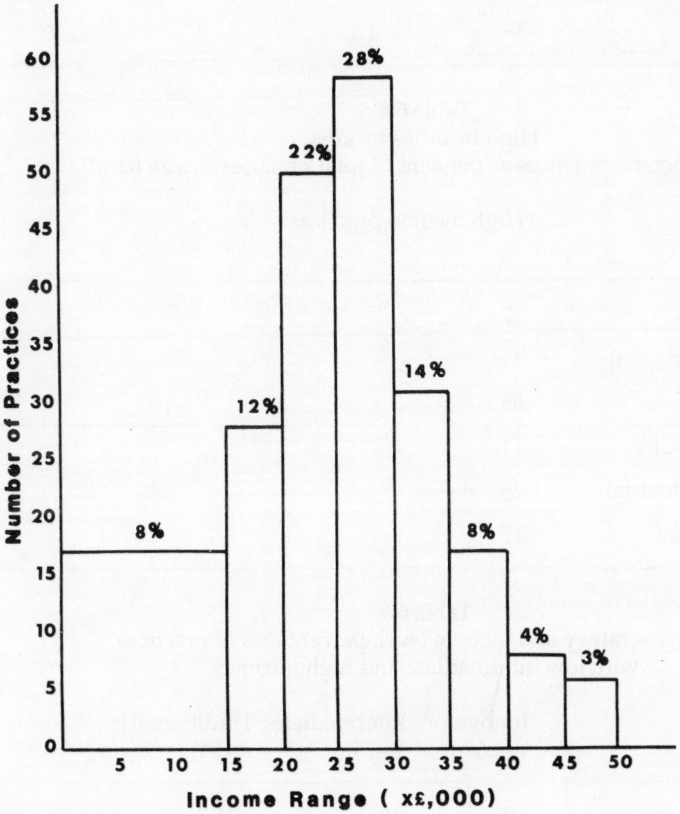

Figure 6.3. Numbers and percentages of practices having specified incomes per partner (full-time equivalent)

Table 6.7
High incomes by partnership size
('High' income practices as per cent of total practices in size band)

Number of partners	High income practices %
2	16
3	15
4	36
5	38
6	44
7+	38

Table 6.8
High incomes by area
('High' income practices as per cent of total practices in size band)

Area	High income practices %
1. NW Suburban	17
4. Thames Valley	31
3. East Rural	55
2. London Inner City	11
5. North East Industrial	26
6. Midlands Urban	17

Table 6.9
Practice strategy and income level: percentages of practices with low intermediate and high incomes

Average net income	Innovator n=86	Intermediate n=75	Traditionalist n=54
Up to £20,000	12	19	39
£20,000-30,000	46	60	43
£30,000+	42	21	18
Total	100	100	100

Premises and capital values

Information was collected on premises and their estimated capital values. Traditionalist practices were often to be found in rented premises, while innovator practices were more likely to own their premises, usually on a collective basis (Table 6.10).

Table 6.10
Ownership of practice premises

	Personally owned		Collectively owned		Rented from health authority		Privately rented		Total number of practices
	%	no	%	no	%	no	%	no	
All practices	19	(50)	40	(104)	29	(75)	12	(30)	259
Innovators	13	(13)	62	(61)	19	(19)	6	(6)	99
Intermediates	19	(17)	33	(30)	32	(29)	16	(14)	90
Traditionalists	29	(20)	19	(13)	39	(27)	14	(10)	70

The capital values of the premises occupied by the innovators were much higher (Table 6.11) than those of intermediates and traditionalists. Capital values were estimated by practices as the market value of the premises, together with the cost of any recent improvement work. Practices lacked accurate information on their own asset values, and these data are more approximate than the income data. Given the differences in the level of property prices between areas, the most relevant comparison is between innovators, intermediates and traditionalists within areas.

Table 6.11
Capital value of premises (£,000)
(For practices owning premises only)

	(1) Innovators	no	(2) Intermediates	no	(3) Traditionalists	no	Ratio of (1):(3)
1. NW Suburban	125.7	(15)	75.1	(7)	47.5	(4)	2.6
3. Thames Valley	183.8	(8)	178.4	(5)	132.0	(5)	1.4
4. East Rural	186.0	(24)	96.5	(4)	44.0	(2)	4.2
2. London Inner City	137.8	(5)	159.2	(6)	65.0	(2)	2.1
5. North East Industrial	139.0	(9)	95.0	(8)	42.3	(4)	3.3
6. Midlands Urban	77.9	(8)	97.8	(12)	49.9	(8)	1.6
7. North Mining	115.0	(7)	43.3	(3)	24.4	(7)	4.7

For premises owned by the practices, the property values were two to three times higher for innovators than for traditionalists, with the exception of the Thames Valley area where all property values were high. However, the differences in capital value per partner were rather less (Table 6.12).

Table 6.12
Capital value of premises per full-time equivalent partner (£,000)

	(1) Innovators	(2) Intermediates	(3) Traditionalists	Ratio of (1):(3)
1. NW Suburban	30.9	21.7	20.8	1.5
3. Thames Valley	41.4	25.9	54.0	0.8
4. East Rural	41.3	32.8	17.9	2.3
2. London Inner City	30.9	21.7	20.8	1.5
5. North East Industrial	27.6	16.0	8.2	3.4
6. Midlands Urban	17.7	26.8	10.6	1.7

The larger average size of innovator practices meant that higher capital values were shared among more partners. Even so the innovators were making much higher investments in their premises. Innovators in the North East Industrial, North Mining and Midlands Urban areas, faced particular risks as it would be a long time before local property prices moved enough to cover the value of the work which had been undertaken.

There were differences in capital values between areas, which reflected local property prices and construction costs, but the high level of capital values for innovators relative to traditionalists was notable in all areas. The innovators appeared to be willing to take on much larger investments even though the risk element was reduced by spreading over a larger number of partners.

Conclusions

The payment system operates nationally in terms of averages for income and costs. The review body sets a target for average net income and practices are reimbursed for some of their costs in relation to the average costs of all practices, established by survey. Such use of averages is designed to produce a fair return to all doctors and to provide an incentive to contain costs.

The survey results show considerable variation in costs and net income. The national payments system interacts with the local environment to bring about higher net incomes in affluent areas with expanding populations, especially for larger practices in such areas. The returns to innovation vary between areas. Practices which invest achieve favourable returns in the more affluent areas, but innovator practices in less affluent areas face higher costs and achieve net incomes which are below the national average. Thus, the payment system does not create incentives for practice development in areas where the need for improved general practice is greatest.

The system is most open to question in relation to the use of an average cost figure. Such a figure is affected by levels of cost among practices in affluent areas. It is very difficult for innovating practices in other areas to cover their costs, especially when they are incurring start-up costs during the early period of practice development. The payment system may provide some incentive to control costs but it does not provide any consistent incentive to improve practice.

7 Services for patients

The study has provided information on services to patients related to different practice strategies. A full discussion of the relationship between patient services and practice types would require data on consultation rates, clinical decision making and outcomes, which have not been collected for this study. However, the present study does provide some information on the provision of clinics and other special sessions for patients.

The evidence showed that innovators organised their practices in distinctive ways. They were more likely to have special clinics, particularly to provide for groups such as diabetics. Innovators were also more likely to offer a complete family planning service, to have an appointments system and an age-sex register, and to have branch surgeries.

1. *Special clinics* Practices have to decide whether to organise special sessions for certain aspects of clinical care. There is no consensus on whether such sessions represent a 'better' or 'worse' way of organising care. Such sessions have been held for a long time for immunisation and family planning but the concept is now being extended to other areas of care. The results of the survey suggest a higher frequency of use of special sessions among innovators. Given the small numbers of positive responses involved, the data are presented by practice type across all areas. Table 7.1 distinguishes practices which have conducted 'special sessions for many years' from those making a 'special effort in consultation'.

Special clinics were very common for antenatal care and immunisation, reflecting a long tradition of holding such clinics. They were also quite common for cervical cytology, babies and well women. However they were much less common for people with diabetes or hypertension, or for geriatric care. For these patients, the majority of doctors preferred to stress special effort in consultations for these conditions, and this was so among innovator as much as among intermediate and traditionalist practices. Special clinics in child health or in women's health usually involved teamwork with a nurse.

Table 7.1

A. Percentages of practices holding special sessions for many years

Type	Total	Innovator	Intermediate	Traditionalist
Antenatal	69	76	69	58
Baby clinic	34	36	39	24
Cervical cytology	38	42	46	20
Immunisation	57	53	68	53
Family planning	29	31	35	15
Well women	18	20	24	9
Diabetes	15	22	13	9
Geriatric	2	3	1	0
Hypertension	11	14	11	5
Other	30	42	29	12

B. Percentages of practices making special effort in consultation

Type	Total	Innovator	Intermediate	Traditionalist
Antenatal	18	15	18	22
Baby clinic	21	17	18	32
Cervical cytology	35	34	26	49
Immunisation	21	20	15	32
Family planning	53	52	54	54
Well women	34	34	31	37
Diabetes	49	43	49	56
Geriatric	58	56	60	58
Hypertension	58	62	52	61
Other	7	7	5	10

The doctors gave their views on the usefulness or otherwise of special sessions. Some doctors were positively against them, particularly for family planning, and the organisation of special sessions would be less useful for small practices. Some gave the impression that perhaps they should have special sessions, but that compelling reasons prevented this. For example, comments ranged from "It is very difficult in a rural area to run special sessions because of transport difficulties and people working", to "we have a definite policy of not having clinics", and "not cost-effective to have special clinics", to one doctor who said there were "not enough women to run an antenatal clinic".

'Other' services (Table 7.1) provided were extremely wide ranging, from flu immunisation and minor surgery, to acupuncture, hypnosis, ear piercing, anxiety clinics, slimming etc. These often reflected the special interest of one partner in a practice.

2. *Maternity services* Doctors were asked whether the practice had had any home confinements in the preceding year. Area 4 (East Rural) accounted for 97 (67 per cent) of the 144 reported home confinements in areas 1-6 for the previous year. The remainder were distributed amongst the other 5 areas, with Area 2 (London Inner City) having only 3 (2 per cent)(see Table 7.2). Most doctors did not favour home confinements. Comments ranged from "too many local problems" "don't feel competent in all eventualities" to "don't believe in them".

Table 7.2
Numbers of home confinements in the previous year

Area	Practices with home confinements %	no	Home confinements %	no
1. NW Suburban	20	(8)	7	(10)
2. London Inner City	4	(1)	2	(3)
3. Thames Valley	13	(4)	6	(8)
4. East Rural	60	(24)	67	(97)
5. NE Industrial	13	(6)	9	(13)
6. Midlands Urban	23	(11)	9	(13)
Total	23	(54)	100	(144)

The numbers of interviewed general practitioners on the obstetric list were analysed by area. Most doctors were on the obstetric list, ranging from 97 per cent in Area 6 (Midlands Urban) to 87 per cent in Area 3 (Thames Valley) the exception being Area 2 (London Inner City) where only 69 per cent of all general practitioners were on the obstetric list. Table 7.3 sets out the number of all doctors and of interviewed doctors on the obstetric list.

Table 7.3
General practitioners on the obstetric list

Area	All doctors on obstetric list		Interviewed doctors on obstetric list	
	%	no	%	no
1. NW Suburban	96	(165)	100	(41)
2. London Inner City	69	(57)	44	(12)
3. Thames Valley	87	(110)	88	(28)
4. East Rural	92	(147)	88	(35)
5. NE Industrial	88	(170)	94	(44)
6. Midlands Urban	100	(149)	98	(47)
7. North Mining	-	-	90	(47)

3. *Family planning services* Doctors were asked how many partners in the practice provided a family planning service and what type the service was. The results are set out in Table 7.4 on an area basis, excluding Area 7. Most doctors said that they would provide a complete service, if patients requested it, though frequently, one partner in a practice would fit IUDs, and other partners would refer patients requiring an IUD to that doctor. Table 7.1 shows that 53 per cent of doctors gave family planning advice during consultations, compared with only 29 per cent who held special sessions. Special sessions were often reserved, either after morning surgery, or as part of a general family planning session. On further analysis it can be seen (Table 7.5) that general practitioners in innovator practices were more likely to provide a complete family planning service.

Table 7.4
Type of family planning service provided by general practitioners in each area

Area	Complete		Pill only		Pill & IUD		All except IUD		All except caps		Total responders
	%	no	%	no	%	no	%	no	%	no	no
1. NW Suburban	45	(78)	23	(39)	6	(10)	18	(31)	8	(14)	172
2. London Inner City	61	(49)	12	(10)	4	(3)	24	(19)	0	(0)	81
3. Thames Valley	64	(80)	1	(1)	1	(1)	32	(40)	2	(3)	125
5. NE Industrial	51	(95)	22	(40)	10	(19)	12	(23)	5	(9)	186
4. East Rural	51	(76)	19	(28)	12	(18)	17	(26)	1	(1)	149
6. Midlands Urban	35	(51)	14	(20)	21	(3)	46	(66)	3	(5)	145

Table 7.5
Provision of a complete family planning service by innovator and other practices

	NW Suburban	London Inner City	Thames Valley	East Rural	NE Industrial	Midlands Urban
	% no	% no	% no	% no	% no	% no
Innovator doctors providing service	59 (51)	68 (26)	78 (38)	54 (61)	43 (29)	39 (16)
Non-innovator doctors providing service	32 (27)	51 (23)	54 (42)	33 (15)	52 (66)	32 (35)
Innovator practices with no complete service	11 (2)	11 (1)	0 (0)	11 (3)	36 (5)	27 (3)
Non-innovator practices with no complete service	32 (7)	22 (4)	24 (5)	46 (6)	33 (11)	54 (20)

4. *Appointment systems* Within most areas, traditionalist practices were much less likely to use appointments systems. For example, in the North Mining area 100 per cent of innovator practices had appointment systems compared to 46 per cent of traditionalist practices (Table 7.6).

Table 7.6
Use of appointment systems by area and practice type

Area	Innovator %	Intermediate %	Traditionalist %	Total %
1. NW Suburban	100	64	63	80
2. London Inner City	67	75	33	63
3. Thames Valley	91	85	63	81
4. East Rural	85	75	80	83
5. NE Industrial	100	95	85	94
6. Midlands Urban	55	72	58	63
7. North Mining	100	83	46	72
Total	87	79	61	77

There were similar differences in practice use of age-sex registers, with 46 per cent of practices in the Midlands Urban area, 67 per cent in the London Inner City and 64 per cent in the North Mining area having such registers, compared with over 75 per cent elsewhere (Table 7.7). However, possession of a register did not imply active use. Many practices did not use such registers regularly.

Table 7.7
Use of age/sex register by area and practice type

Area	Innovator %	Intermediate %	Traditionalist %	Total %
1. NW Suburban	100*	64	63	80
2. London Inner City	100	58	33	67
3. Thames Valley	100	77	38	75
4. East Rural	96	88	40	88
5. NE Industrial	86	85	54	77
6. Midlands Urban	73	50	26	46
7. North Mining	75	50	64	64
Total	92	68	44	74

* 100% of innovator practices in NW Suburban have age/sex registers.

5. *Provision of branch premises* Innovator practices were found to be more likely than others to have branch premises (see Table 7.8). This would seem to reflect the larger size of innovator practices, servicing larger numbers of patients.

Table 7.8
Practices which have branches by practice type

Type	One surgery only %	At least one branch %
Innovators	54	47
Intermediates	67	33
Traditionalists	63	37
All	61	39

6. *Immunisation information* Comparatively few practices received information on the percentage of children immunised in their practices, but there were differences depending on practice type. Thirty-nine per cent of innovators, 36 per cent of intermediates, but only 25 per cent of traditionalists received such information. This excludes Area 7.

Conclusions

With differences in strategy have come differences in practice style and organisation. Innovators were more likely to hold special clinics and to have introduced a team approach, and they were also more likely to have regular information about immunisation. Improvements in practice structure seemed to lead to an expansion in the range of services offered and to a more comprehensive service.

8 Practice organisation and views of the future

The previous chapters described the results of the survey relating practice structure to practice strategy. This chapter looks at the views of the doctors on the current state of their practices and on future prospects.

The professional and personal characteristics of the doctors interviewed are set out in Table 8.1. As described in Chapter 3, one partner from each practice was interviewed in areas 1-6. In area 7, a postal questionnaire was used and 55 per cent of all general practitioners responded. Results from this latter area therefore represent the views of a larger proportion of doctors than those of the other six areas. Table 8.1 shows significant differences between types of practice. Doctors in the innovator practices were more likely to have post-graduate qualifications and much more likely to be members of the Royal College of General Practitioners.

The doctors interviewed were often the most senior in the practices. The survey covered 70-80 per cent of practices in each area but the interviewed doctors were not necessarily representative in their personal views. However, the results are indicative of how a large group of family doctors sees the future of general practice (Tables 8.1 and 8.2.) Even so, the selection does not do full justice to the views of certain important minorities among general practitioners such as female and Asian doctors, since they were rarely the doctors interviewed.

The average age of the interviewed doctors was higher than that of the average for all the doctors in the study. For the interviewed doctors, average ages were 46, 48 and 47 years for innovators, intermediates and traditionalists respectively. Corresponding ages for *all* doctors were 42, 44 and 45 years. These figures all exclude area 7. The age differences reflect the fact that senior partners were more frequently interviewed.

Female doctors were under represented in the interview sample. Only 7 per cent of those interviewed were female (Areas 1-6) whereas in these 6 areas, female doctors were 17.5 per cent of all doctors.

Table 8.1

Personal characteristics of the interviewed doctors in each practice category

(Interviewed doctors only)

	Innovators		Intermediates		Traditionalists		Total	
Professional characteristics	%	no	%	no	%	no	%	no
Doctors with post graduate qualifications*	75	(68)	54	(46)	54	(32)	62	(146)
Doctors with MRCGP (inc Area 7)	47	(53)	28	(27)	21	(16)	33	(96)
Doctors with BMA membership (inc Area 7)	80	(90)	81	(79)	70	(53)	77	(222)
Average age (years)*	46		48		47		-	
Sex male*	96	(87)	91	(77)	92	(54)	-	
female*	4	(4)	9	(8)	9	(5)	-	
Ethnic or national background								
British	44	(88)	33	(67)	23	(47)		(202)
Asian	16	(5)	34	(11)	50	(16)		(32)
Irish	14	(1)	29	(2)	57	(4)		(7)
Other	13	(2)	69	(11)	19	(3)		(16)

* Area 7 excluded.

Attitudes to general practice

1. *Views on fee for service* How far were views on the payment system dependent on the strategy adopted by practices? 54 per cent of all general practitioners thought that the principle of fee for service should be extended to other areas, (Table 8.3), the proportion being slightly higher in the innovator practices (60 per cent) than in the intermediates (52 per cent) and the traditionalists (49 per cent). Female partners were rather more likely to want to phase out fee for service (24 per cent, as against 9 per cent for male general practitioners). Comments by doctors on fee for service were numerous and included "the more like a commercial business the better the system would be!" and "there should really be different ways of funding to encourage work to be done". There was also some ambivalence; "the principle is sound, but shouldn't,

Table 8.2
Total number of doctors in each study area, and number of doctors interviewed in each area

Area	Interviewed doctors %	Interviewed doctors no	Total number of doctors
1. NW Suburban	24	41	172
2. London Inner City	33	27	83
3. Thames Valley	25	32	127
4. East Rural	25	40	159
5. NE Industrial	24	47	193
6. Midlands Urban	32	48	149
7. North Mining*	60	52	87
Total	30	287	970

* Pilot study area.

if extended, reduce doctors' basic income". A few had reservations; "morally a bad idea - practically is an incentive for areas that need looking at anyway". Procedures favoured by family doctors for inclusion in the fee for service options were numerous. Most favoured were an extension of cervical cytology tests to younger women, minor surgery, paediatric surveillance, and all kinds of screening. Some doctors even mentioned out of hours calls, home visits and blood tests.

2. *Views on list size* Only 9 per cent of the general practitoners in innovator practices felt that it was very important to have a large list in order to maintain a reasonably high income, but this figure rose to 13 per cent of the doctors in intermediate practices and to 16 per cent of those in traditionalist practices (Table 8.3). 77 per cent of doctors across areas felt that it was better to have a list of average size and to develop income from fees for service. Some doctors found it difficult to decide between the two options presented. The overall trend was for a higher proportion of doctors in traditionalist practices to favour a large list and hence obtain income from capitation rather than by fee for service. According to one doctor "there should be a balance between the two - the elderly might be "left out" if there was too much emphasis on fees for service", and another commented that "doctors should be paid a fair sum for a good job without financial incentives for doing what they should do anyway".

3. *Views on pressure of work* General practitioners were asked whether they could cope within their normal working hours in most weeks. One doctor asked "what are

normal working hours?" The question had been phrased in this way to allow the doctors themselves to interpret the question in their own way. Overall, 45 per cent of doctors felt that they could cope, the figure varying from 50 per cent in innovator practices, to 44 per cent in intermediates and only 41 per cent in traditionalist practices. (Table 8.3). Conversely, 43 per cent of doctors in innovator practices, 42 per cent in intermediates, but 48 per cent in traditionalist practices felt under some pressure. However, one doctor felt that "it is a myth about pressure; you organise your life to cope and to enjoy it", and another commented, "a doctor makes his own workload. A caring doctor will always be under pressure".

4. *Intentions about desire for change or improvement* 57 per cent of general practitioners in all types of practices hoped to bring about major changes and improvements in services over the next three years (Table 8.3).

But, as one doctor commented, "An older doctor near to retirement age might agree that his services offered were about right, but not younger doctors".

Table 8.3
Responses of doctors in the 3 practice categories to statements about general practice

	Total n=287	Innovator n=113	Intermediate n=98	Traditionalist n=76
Agreeing that:	% no	% no	% no	% no
The principle of fee for items of service should be extended to other areas	54 (156)	60 (68)	52 (51)	49 (37)
It is very important to have a large list (of patients) in order to maintain a reasonably high income	12 (35)	9 (10)	13 (13)	16 (12)
It is better to have a list of average size and to develop income from fees for service	77 (221)	83 (94)	74 (72)	72 (55)
I would hope to bring about major change and improvements in services over the next 3 years	57 (164)	59 (67)	54 (53)	58 (44)
I can cope within normal working hours in most weeks	45 (130)	50 (56)	44 (43)	41 (31)
I am sometimes under pressure to complete all that needs doing in a week	44 (126)	43 (49)	42 (41)	47 (36)

Area 7 included in all cases.

Attitudes to general practice analysed by area

When the same questions on the payment system and workload were analysed on an area basis, some greater differences emerged (Table 8.4).

1. *Fee for service* Most general practitioners, in all study areas thought that the principle of fee for service should be extended to other service areas (57 per cent) but only 41 per cent of doctors in Area 2 (London Inner City) and 45 per cent of doctors in Area 5 (NE Industrial) held this view. Twenty-nine per cent felt that the present system was satisfactory, rising from 17 per cent in Area 1 to 36 per cent in Area 5. Overall, only 10 per cent of interviewed doctors felt that fee for service was a bad system and should be phased out, but 22 per cent of doctors in Area 2 did hold this view, possibly reflecting the fact that inner city doctors have difficulty in contacting patients to provide the services which attract a fee, and would hence favour its abolition.

Table 8.4
Response of the interviewed doctors to certain questions about general practice, analysed by area

	NW Suburban		Thames Valley		East Rural		London Inner City		NE Industrial		Midlands Urban	
Agreeing that:	%	no	%	no	%	no	%	no	%	no	%	no
Fee for service												
The principle should be extended to other areas	73	(30)	72	(23)	58	(23)	41	(11)	45	(21)	52	(25)
The present system is satisfactory	17	(7)	19	(6)	35	(14)	33	(9)	36	(17)	31	(15)
The principle is a bad one and should be phased out	7	(3)	9	(3)	3	(1)	22	(6)	13	(6)	10	(5)
Don't know	2	(1)	0	-	5	(2)	4	(1)	6	(3)	6	(3)
List size												
Important to have large list to maintain reasonably high income	5	(2)	9	(3)	8	(3)	11	(3)	11	(5)	13	(6)
Better to have average list and develop income from fee for service	85	(35)	72	(23)	75	(30)	78	(21)	79	(37)	77	(37)
Don't know	10	(4)	19	(6)	18	(7)	11	(3)	11	(5)	10	(5)

(Table continued...)

Agreeing that:	NW Suburban %	no	Thames Valley %	no	East Rural %	no	London Inner City %	no	NE Industrial %	no	Midlands Urban %	no
Workload												
I can cope within my normal hours in most weeks	54	(22)	19	(6)	48	(19)	44	(12)	51	(24)	38	(18)
Sometimes under pressure to complete all that needs doing in a week	32	(13)	63	(20)	45	(18)	41	(11)	38	(18)	52	(25)
Under great pressure and constantly short of time	15	(6)	19	(6)	8	(3)	15	(4)	11	(5)	10	(5)
Services												
Our services are about right & we don't expect to make changes	34	(14)	34	(11)	55	(22)	37	(10)	38	(18)	46	(22)
Hope to make major changes and improvements	59	(24)	66	(21)	45	(18)	63	(17)	62	(29)	54	(26)
Neither	7	(3)	0	-	0	-	0	-	0	-	0	-

2. *List size* In all areas, general practitioners favoured a list of average size. There were no great differences. Variations in list size have ceased to be a live issue for general practitioners (Table 8.4).

3. *Pressure of work* When asked about their workload, 43 per cent over all areas felt that they could cope, though this fell to only 19 per cent in Area 3 (Thames Valley). But upon further analysis the low figure was found to be attributable to the urban part of this area and views in the other more typically affluent suburban parts of this area were much more in line with the average figures. A minority (12 per cent) of doctors in all areas felt under "great pressure", the figure rising from only 8 per cent in Area 4 (East Rural) to 19 per cent in Area 3 (Thames Valley).There were no clear differences between the less affluent areas and the others in doctors perceptions of workload.

4. *Desire for change or improvement* When asked whether they intended to make changes and improvements to their services, 57 per cent said they hoped to do so. The lowest figure (45 per cent) for Area 4 (East Rural) may reflect the already good facilities in the practices in this area.

5. *Policy on home visits* The overwhelming majority of general practitioners (75 per cent) were happy with the number of home visits they were making. Only Area 5 (NE Industrial) showed any variation from this pattern, with only 55 per cent happy with the present situation and 28 per cent who wanted to reduce home visits, a much higher percentage than in any of the other 5 areas (Table 8.5). Traditionalist practices were more likely than others to want to reduce their home visits.

The pressure of home visits seemed to be a major issue for family doctors at the time of the earlier surveys, especially that of Cartwright in 1964 (Cartwright, 1967). Even in 1986, the Workload Study showed that home visits were taking up an average of 9.81 hours a week, or 28 per cent of total working time (Department of Health and Social Security, 1987b). But, in general, there does not seem to be much discontent with the level of home visiting except among traditionalist practices in the older industrial areas. In a few areas there is still a traditional social pressure for high levels of home visiting, but in most other areas this pressure now seems to be diminished.

Table 8.5
How would you describe your personal policy on making home visits?

	NW Suburban		London Inner City		Thames Valley		East Rural		NE Industrial		Midlands Urban		Total	
	%	no	%	no	%	no	%	no	%	no	%	no	%	no
I am ready to make home visits and am prepared to see more time devoted to them in the future	2	(1)	4	(1)	9	(3)	3	(1)	6	(3)	10	(5)	6	(14)
I am happy with the number of home visits I make	80	(33)	81	(22)	78	(25)	90	(36)	55	(26)	73	(35)	75	(177)
I am keen to reduce the number of home visits & replace them with other forms of service, eg phone consultations	7	(3)	15	(4)	6	(2)	5	(2)	28	(13)	15	(7)	13	(31)
Other	10	(4)	0	-	6	(2)	3	(1)	11	(5)	2	(1)	6	(13)
Total		(41)		(27)		(32)		(40)		(47)		(48)		(235)

Attitude to general practice analysed by age of the doctor

There was little difference in general practitioner attitudes to list size when analyzed by the age of the doctor. The overwhelming preference at all ages was for an average list size. Similar results were obtained when views on fee for service were analysed by age. However, there was an age effect with workload. Older doctors felt under less pressure than younger ones (Table 8.6). Thirty-seven per cent of doctors under 40 felt that they could cope within normal working hours, rising to 68 per cent of 60-69 year olds. An additional 51 per cent of the under 40s felt under some pressure but only 16 per cent of the 60-69 year olds felt that way. However, 16 per cent of the older group felt "hard pressed" compared with 13 per cent of the younger group. Overall, 67 per cent of doctors under 50, but only 32 per cent of the 60-69 year olds felt under some or great pressure.

Table 8.6
Attitude of interviewed doctors to workload, by age.

	Under 40	Under 49	40-49	50-59	60-69	70+	60+
	% no	% no	% no	% no	% no	% no	% no
I can cope within my normal working hours	37 (23)	33 (46)	30 (23)	53 (34)	68 (17)	75 (3)	69 (20)
I am sometimes under pressure	51 (32)	55 (78)	59 (46)	34 (22)	16 (4)	25 (1)	17 (5)
I am under great pressure and continually short of time	13 (8)	12 (17)	12 (9)	13 (8)	16 (4)	0 -	14 (4)
No response	- (1)	0 -	0 -	0 -	0 -	0 -	0 -
No. doctors	(64)	(141)	(78)	(64)	(25)	(4)	(29)

Attitude to general practice analysed by country of birth of the doctor

When analysed by country of birth of responding doctor, Asians were found to be slightly more in favour of the principle of fee for service being extended to other areas (72 per cent, against 56 per cent of British born doctors). Slightly more were under great workload pressure (24 per cent, against 11 per cent of British born doctors), but numbers of Asians questioned were small.

Practice organisation

1. *Records* The doctors were asked several questions about the way in which their practices were organised and whether they considered this organisation to be satisfactory. They were asked whether they considered the administration and organisation of their practice records to be very satisfactory, adequate, sometimes inadequate or nearly always inadequate (Table 8.7). On an area basis, 28 per cent of practices felt that their situation was very satisfactory, with most practices (47 per cent) agreeing their records were adequate. A sizable minority (24 per cent) felt that organisation of their records was sometimes inadequate, though very few (2 per cent) felt them to be nearly always inadequate. Considerable effort seems to have been made in some practices to improve records, as some doctors commented: "the last two years have been spent summarising"; "records have been ruthlessly pruned"; "clearing out ghost patients", was also mentioned. Of course, the possession of adequate records is a prerequisite for becoming a training practice, which could account for some of this activity.

Table 8.7

Responses of individual doctors when asked whether they considered the organisation of their records to be satisfactory

	Organisation of records								
	Very satisfactory		Adequate		Sometimes inadequate		Nearly always inadequate		Total
Area	%	no	%	no	%	no	%	no	no
1. NW Suburban	38	(15)	35	(14)	25	(10)	3	(1)	(40)
2. London Inner City	30	(8)	56	(15)	15	(4)	0	-	(27)
3. Thames Valley	29	(9)	52	(16)	19	(6)	0	-	(31)
5. NE Industrial	26	(12)	43	(20)	28	(13)	4	(2)	(47)
6. Midlands Urban	23	(11)	53	(25)	23	(11)	0	-	(47)
4. East Rural	23	(9)	48	(19)	28	(11)	3	(1)	(40)
Total	28	(64)	47	(109)	24	(55)	2	(4)	(232)

When analysed by practice types, a higher percentage of general practitioners in innovator practices were likely to consider their records to be very satisfactory or adequate (77 per cent in innovator practices, 67 per cent in intermediate and 61 per cent traditionalist practices). Nevertheless, when asked whetherthey had any plans to improve the administration and organisation of their records in the next three years, those most intent on improvement were the doctors in innovator practices (Table 8.8).

Table 8.8

Doctors who said that they would like to improve the administration of their records

Area	Total %	Total no	Innovators %	Innovators no	Intermediates %	Intermediates no	Traditionalists %	Traditionalists no
4. East Rural	80	(32)	82	(22)	75	(6)	80	(4)
5. NE Industrial	75	(35)	93	(13)	70	(14)	62	(8)
3. Thames Valley	72	(23)	73	(8)	69	(9)	75	(6)
1. NW Suburban	66	(27)	63	(12)	71	(10)	63	(5)
6. Midlands Urban	63	(30)	64	(7)	72	(13)	53	(10)
2. London Inner City	59	(16)	89	(8)	42	(5)	50	(3)
Total	69	(163)	77	(70)	67	(57)	61	(36)

2. *Staffing* In terms of staffing, general practitioners were asked how they would describe the level of secretarial/administrative staff employed by their practice and whether, if they considered staffing levels to be inadequate, they had any plans for extra staff. Comments on staffing ranged from "excellent", to "would crumble without YTS girls" to "staff are a bunch of idiots!" The results (Table 8.9) indicated that most (84 per cent) of the doctors considered their staffing level to be either always or usually adequate, but 25 per cent of general practitioners in Area 6 (Midlands Urban) described the situation as "frequently inadequate". The general impression was that although doctors in innovator practices had better organised practices, they were still more likely to be looking for improvements than were doctors in the other two types of practices.

In addition, questions were asked about the adequacy or inadequacy of the service available from District Health Authority employed staff, particularly district nurses, health visitors and midwives. In general, satisfaction was high, particularly in the rural area (Area 4) and particularly with midwives. Satisfaction was lowest in the more urban areas, particularly Area 6 (Midlands Urban) (see Table 8.10). For Area 7 (N Mining), all doctors were asked in the postal questionnaire about District Health Authority employed staff. Here, 78 per cent of respondents felt the district nursing service was adequate, 84 per cent the health visiting service, and 96 per cent the midwifery service. These figures have been excluded from Table 8.10.

Overall, 65 per cent of practices in Areas 1-6 felt that additional staffing was required. The list of extra staff mentioned was extensive and included physiotherapists, psychologists, social workers, counsellors of all kinds, health educators and chiropodists. Secretaries, receptionists, clerks, computer operators, etc were needed to help with managing the practice.

Table 8.9
Responses of individual general practitioners as to whether they personally considered their secretarial/administrative staffing to be satisfactory

Area	Secretarial/administrative staff: Always adequate % no	Usually adequate % no	Frequently inadequate % no	Nearly always inadequate % no	Total responses no
1. NW Suburban	50 (20)	40 (16)	8 (3)	3 (1)	(40)
7. North Mining	35 (18)	52 (27)	12 (6)	2 (1)	(52)
5. NE Industrial	34 (16)	53 (25)	11 (5)	2 (1)	(47)
2. London Inner City	26 (7)	63 (17)	7 (2)	4 (1)	(27)
4. East Rural	25 (10)	58 (23)	13 (5)	5 (2)	(40)
3. Thames Valley	22 (7)	66 (21)	13 (4)	0 -	(32)
6. Midlands Urban	42 (2)	67 (32)	25 (12)	42 (2)	(48)
Total	28 (80)	56 (161)	13 (37)	3 (8)	(286)

Table 8.10
How would you describe the service available to your patients from District Health Authority employed staff?

Area	Doctors agreeing service is adequate: District nurses % no	Health visitors % no	Midwives % no	Responding doctors no
1. NW Suburban	93 (37)	75 (30)	80 (32)	(40)
2. London Inner City	67 (18)	70 (19)	78 (21)	(27)
3. Thames Valley	72 (23)	75 (24)	72 (23)	(32)
4. East Rural	73 (29)	70 (28)	90 (36)	(40)
5. NE Industrial	79 (37)	68 (32)	87 (41)	(47)
6. Midlands Urban	56 (27)	65 (31)	65 (31)	(48)
Total	73 (171)	70 (164)	79 (184)	(234)

3. *Premises* The doctors were asked for their views on their main practice premises. Overall, 74 per cent of doctors interviewed were either very satisfied, or fairly satisfied with their main practice premises (Table 8.11), but as one doctor commented "you can always see something that needs doing". Only 20 per cent were dissatisfied, but this rose to 41 per cent in Area 3 (Thames Valley), most of the dissatisfaction being in the urban parts of the area. Interestingly, in the London Inner City area (Area 2), 71 per cent of doctors were either very or fairly satisfied with their premises, but 15 per cent were very dissatisfied, as against an average for all areas of only 6 per cent. The overall high level of satisfaction in this area may reflect the difficulty experienced in persuading doctors to take part in the survey, and the fact that those who did were thought to be those in the better located premises. Family doctors in innovator practices were much more likely to be satisfied with their premises, wherever they were located.

Table 8.11
Satisfaction with main practice premises

Area	Very satisfied % no	Fairly satisfied % no	Dissatisfied % no	Very dissatisfied % no	Total responders no
4. East Rural	50 (20)	30 (12)	20 (8)	0 -	(40)
5. NE Industrial	40 (19)	30 (14)	19 (9)	11 (5)	(47)
1. NW Suburban	39 (16)	39 (16)	22 (9)	0 -	(41)
6. Midlands Urban	31 (15)	50 (24)	13 (6)	6 (3)	(48)
2. London Inner City	30 (8)	41 (11)	15 (4)	15 (4)	(27)
7. North Mining	27 (14)	54 (28)	15 (8)	4 (2)	(52)
3. Thames Valley	19 (6)	28 (9)	41 (13)	13 (4)	(32)
Total	34 (98)	40 (114)	20 (57)	6 (18)	(287)

Satisfaction with premises was analysed according to ownership and the results are set out in Table 8.12. Across all areas, doctors in collectively owned premises were the most likely to be very satisfied (46 per cent) and those in premises rented from the health authority were most likely to be dissatisfied. Those in privately rented accommodation were the most likely of all to be dissatisfied. As one doctor said, probably summing up the views of many in health centres "I would prefer not to be in premises owned by the health authority. If younger I would consider building under the cost rent scheme", and another commented "I cannot improve anything until I own my own premises".

Table 8.12

Satisfaction with premises depending on type of ownership.

Ownership	Very satisfied % no	Fairly satisfied % no	Dissatisfied % no	Very dissatisfied % no
Collectively owned	46 (44)	29 (28)	20 (19)	5 (5)
Personally owned	26 (11)	56 (24)	14 (6)	5 (2)
Rented from Health Authority	37 (24)	32 (21)	22 (14)	9 (6)
Privately rented	13 (4)	43 (13)	33 (10)	10 (3)
Other	100 (1)	0 -	0 -	0 -

(Excludes Area 7)

The aggregated responses for all interviewed doctors were analysed according to whether they had had a major extension in the past five years costing more than £3000. Of the 112 practices which had had a major extension (Table 8.13) 46 per cent were very satisfied and a further 39 per cent were fairly satisfied. (Table 8.14). Those doctors in practices which had not had an extension were more likely to be dissatisfied. (Forty-one per cent dissatisfied or very dissatisfied against only 15 per cent in premises which had been extended).

Table 8.13

Practices having any major extension or modernisation in the past 5 years

Area	Total % no	Innovators % no	Intermediates % no	Traditionalists % no
2. London Inner City	63 (17)	78 (7)	75 (9)	17 (1)
4. East Rural	63 (25)	78 (21)	25 (2)	40 (2)
1. NW Suburban	54 (22)	74 (14)	36 (5)	38 (3)
6. Midlands Urban	42 (20)	64 (7)	44 (8)	26 (5)
5. NE Industrial	40 (19)	64 (9)	40 (8)	15 (2)
3. Thames Valley	28 (9)	55 (6)	8 (1)	25 (2)
Total	48 (112)	57 (64)	29 (33)	13 (15)

Table 8.14
Satisfaction with premises and whether there has been a major extension within the past 5 years

	Major extension		No major extension		Total
	%	no	%	no	no
Very satisfied	46*	(52)	25	(31)	(83)
Fairly satisfied	39	(44)	34	(42)	(86)
Dissatisfied	13	(14)	29	(35)	(49)
Very dissatisfied	2	(2)	12	(14)	(16)
Total		(112)		(122)	(234)

(Area 7 excluded)

* of the 112 practices which had a major extension, 46 per cent were very satisfied.

Doctors were asked whether they would like to move, or to extend or modernise their practices. Overall, 38 per cent were happy where they were, but 16 per cent wanted to move, 25 per cent wanted an extension, and 11 per cent a modernisation (Table 8.15). Doctors in the East Rural and NE Industrial areas were the least likely to want any changes while those in the Thames Valley, London Inner City and North Mining areas were most dissatisfied with the existing situation.

Table 8.15
Do you personally want to see any of the following alternatives for your practice?

	Move		Extension		Modernisation		Other		None/NA		Total
Area	%	no	%	no	%	no	%	no	%	no	no
7. N Mining	26	(11)	14	(6)	26	(11)	16	(7)	19	(8)	(43)
2. London Inner City	19	(5)	39	(10)	0	-	4	(1)	39	(10)	(26)
3. Thames Valley	19	(6)	41	(13)	13	(4)	3	(1)	25	(8)	(32)
5. NE Industrial	15	(7)	11	(5)	15	(7)	11	(5)	49	(23)	(47)
6. Midlands Urban	15	(7)	28	(13)	13	(6)	9	(4)	36	(17)	(47)
1. NW Suburban	10	(4)	26	(10)	0	-	15	(6)	49	(19)	(39)
4. East Rural	8	(3)	30	(11)	3	(1)	8	(3)	51	(19)	(37)
Total	16	(43)	25	(68)	11	(29)	10	(27)	38	(104)	(271)

Table 8.16 compares satisfaction with premises, with whether the doctors wanted to move or to extend or modernise their premises. Of those who were very satisfied with their premises, only 1 per cent wanted to move, but this figure rose to 69 per cent of doctors who were very dissatisfied with their premises.

Table 8.16
Satisfaction with premises and whether general practitioners want to see premises altered

	Move	Extension	Modernise	Other	None/NA
	% no	% no	% no	% no	% no
Very satisfied	*1 (1)	15 (12)	4 (3)	6 (5)	74 (59)
Fairly satisfied	6 (5)	30 (26)	11 (9)	9 (8)	44 (37)
Dissatisfied	31 (15)	48 (23)	6 (3)	15 (7)	0 -
Very dissatisfied	69 (11)	6 (1)	19 (3)	6 (1)	0 -

* Of those who were very satisfied with their premises, 1 per cent wanted to move.

Views about the future

General Practitioners were asked for their personal views about how they felt their practices might change in the future in response to pressure of work, income, partnership size and list size. Most doctors expected pressure of work to increase (55 per cent) (Table 8.17), with doctors from innovator practices more likely to express this view (61 per cent). Most (59 per cent) also thought that real incomes would rise although again doctors in innovator practices were more likely to expect this to happen (66 per cent), than doctors in traditionalist practices (51 per cent) (Table 8.18). From Table 8.19, it can be seen that only one in five doctors expected their number of partners to increase. Three quarters thought that their partnership size would remain the same. Perhaps the most surprising result concerned views on future list size (Table 8.20). Forty-four per cent of interviewed general practitioners thought that list size would be larger in three years' time, and only 7 per cent thought it would be lower. However, it is likely that the question had been interpreted as referring to the practice list size as a whole, which could well be expected to rise in areas of expanding population. These practices might well then take on another partner which would mean an overall fall in personal list size. Several doctors remarked that patient expectations were rising and one commented that there was now "more work produced by the same number of patients". Another view was that "People's expectations are rising beyond what you can provide, and there will be more preventive care."

Table 8.17
Doctors' views on whether pressure of work is likely to be higher, lower or the same in three years time

	Higher	Lower	Same	Total
Practice type	% no	% no	% no	no
All Innovators	61 (54)	7 (6)	33 (29)	(89)
All Intermediates	52 (44)	12 (10)	37 (31)	(85)
All Traditionalists	52 (30)	12 (7)	36 (21)	(58)
All practices	55 (128)	10 (23)	35 (81)	(232)

Table 8.18
Doctors' views on whether their income is likely to be higher, lower or the same in three years time

	Higher	Lower	Same	Total
Practice type	% no	% no	% no	no
All Innovators	66 (59)	7 (6)	27 (24)	(89)
All Intermediates	58 (48)	11 (9)	31 (26)	(83)
All Traditionalists	51 (30)	7 (4)	42 (25)	(59)
All practices	59 (137)	8 (19)	33 (75)	(231)

Table 8.19
Doctors views on whether their number of partners is likely to have become higher, lower or stayed the same in three years time

	Higher	Lower	Same	Total
Practice type	% no	% no	% no	no
All Innovators	19 (17)	3 (3)	78 (70)	(90)
All Intermediates	26 (22)	1 (1)	73 (61)	(84)
All Traditionalists	20 (12)	3 (2)	76 (45)	(59)
All practices	22 (51)	3 (6)	76 (176)	(233)

Table 8.20
Doctors' views on whether their list size is likely to have become higher, lower or stayed the same in three years time

Practice type	Higher %	Higher no	Lower %	Lower no	Same %	Same no	Total no
All Innovators	49	(44)	6	(5)	46	(41)	(90)
All Intermediates	42	(35)	10	(8)	49	(41)	(84)
All Traditionalists	39	(23)	7	(4)	54	(32)	(59)
All practices	44	(102)	7	(17)	49	(114)	(233)

Summary

The survey has shown distinct differences in practice strategy. The evidence from the interviews with the doctors themselves allows some tentative conclusions on whether these differences in strategy were related to distinctive attitudes. In general, most family doctors in the survey showed support for the principle of a closer link between pay and work actually done. There was little opposition to the extension of fee for service. Innovators were more likely to stress the importance of fee for service income whilst traditionalists were more likely to think in terms of higher list size as the best way of increasing income. Innovators were also more inclined to be looking for major improvements in their practices over the next few years.

The level of satisfaction with premises and staffing was reasonably high. The greatest concern was in relation to practice records and here the level of concern expressed by innovators was higher than that of doctors in other types of practice. In general, the survey showed a low level of concern about excessive workload, and all groups were equally likely to expect increased workload as well as increased income in the future.

The evidence on practice decisions had suggested that there was a distinctive group of general practitioners which had implemented a strategy of innovation. The evidence on opinions provides further evidence of the distinct identity of this group, and of the contrast between the innovators and the traditionalists. The evidence also showed that the principle of linking pay to work actually done found favour among family doctors. The results showed that family doctors were more concerned about improving their practice records, and that deficiencies in premises and staffing were of less immediate concern.

9 Conclusions and policy implications

The model (Figure 1.1) set out a framework for analysing the decisions made by family doctors. Decisions on practice structure and strategy might be influenced by the personal characteristics of the partners; by the impact of the payment system at the local level; and by the environment surrounding the practice. These decisions in turn lead to results defined in the model as outcomes for partners and services for patients.

'General Practice' has often been seen as an entity which changes in a consistent way over a period of time (British Medical Association, 1984). The aim of the model was to suggest an alternative approach. Practices can be defined as 'firms' working within a certain territory, and the aggregate trends sum up the disparate decisions made by these 'firms'. A *description* of the trends cannot explain very much about the *causation* of changes; nor does it explain the variability in practice response.

Partnerships are already economic agents making decisions in a local market. Practices have had increasing discretion within the policy framework set by the Family Doctor Charter. Their use of this discretion may help to show how partnerships would react in a more developed system of internal markets. Partnerships have already had useful (although subsidised) training in the skills required for such a market, including raising capital in private markets and acting as employers.

The study does not deal with some of the most important aspects of general practice, such as the quality of care to patients and no data were collected on clinical decisions or on outcomes. This is a study of one aspect of general practice, but the quality of decision-making described here may give some guide to decision-making on patient care and treatment. For example, a practice that spends time and effort on improving its premises, on taking part in the vocational training scheme, and on establishing teamwork between family doctors and nursing staff may or may not be practising good medicine, but it has made commitments which suggest an aspiration towards improved care, and it has established networks which potentially lay its decisions open to some scrutiny. In the case of participation in the training scheme and employment of a practice nurse, the links between these decisions and good clinical practice are a little more than circumstantial. Practices which take part in the vocational training scheme are showing that they are prepared to have an external audit of the practice by their peers, and doctors who work in a team with nurses are also open to scrutiny and are willing to undertake a wider range of tasks (Cartwright and Anderson, 1981). Thus certain decisions on 'inputs' can be taken as pointers to practice service mix in other respects. Practices which take part in the training scheme, invest in premises and employ nurses, can fairly be labelled as 'innovators'. Practices are now under pressure to develop new services in prevention. (Department of Health and Social Security, 1987). The study did not collect evidence directly on practice intentions nor on the willingness of practices to respond in what was described in Chapter 2 as the fourth phase of primary care, but the decisions on practice structure may give some guide to the management capability of practices in the face of these new demands. Thus, an 'innovator' practice is 'better' than a traditional practice, in terms of its likely management ability to adapt to new demands.

In Chapter 1 certain variables were put forward as likely to be important in influencing decisions on strategy, and certain hypotheses were presented on the possible effects of variables such as age and area. The main results relating to the variables in Table 1.1 can be summarised as follows:

1. *Age* It was expected that age would be a major factor affecting practice decisions - that such decisions would show a life cycle effect so that younger doctors would 'invest' in new premises and adapt to new methods. Such life cycle effects were found in some urban areas (London Inner City, Midlands Urban, North Mining, Table 4.1) where there were high proportions of practices with an average partnership age greater than 50, but the results suggest that the life cycle effect is now becoming much weaker. Larger practices are now more common. They have partners of different ages and such practices have an existence independent of the career ageing of the individual partners.

2. *Sex* About a half of general practice partnerships had at least one female partner, with the lowest proportions in the North Mining (32 per cent) and the East Rural (30 per cent) areas (Table 4.2). Overall, only 36 per cent of traditionalist practices had at least one female partner, but the figure for innovators and intermediates averaged 55 per cent (Table 5.8). These differences may have been a factor in the finding that well women clinics were more often present in innovator and intermediate practices (22 per cent) compared with traditionalist practices (9 per cent) (Table 7.1). It is impossible to tell from the study findings whether female doctors set up the well women clinics, or whether female doctors were attracted to practices already possessing such clinics, but there may be a link. Apart from this however, the presence or absence of a female partner had little effect on practice services.

3. *Ethnic background* There was considerable area variability in the distribution of Asian doctors. 60 per cent of practices in the North Mining area had at least one Asian partner compared to only 3 per cent of practices in the East Rural area (Table 4.3). Asian partners were to be found mainly in areas with lower than average net income per partner, and within those areas, practices with Asian partners were likely to have lower incomes and to be in non-innovating practices. 62 per cent of practices with low net incomes (under £20,000 a year per partner) had Asian partners. The system is currently working so that Asian doctors are less willing or less able to invest, and face lower incomes than other family doctors. They are also more restricted in the choice of areas in which they practice, with a higher chance of location in poorer inner city areas.

4. *Length of service* It was expected that the variable would be significantly related to practice decisions, an expectation based on many studies of the labour market, where labour turnover and amounts of job training are significantly related to length of service (Rees and Shultz, 1970). As with age, the increased size of practices is leading to a greater similarity in average length of service of partners. The survey results were negative in that the average length of service of partners was similar across all areas and practice types.

5. *Nature of the contract* Apart from a few male family doctors in their 50s, part-time contracts were confined to female doctors. 39 per cent of female doctors in the survey were working on a part-time basis. There would appear to be a division growing up between full-time male doctors on the one hand and the many female doctors who work on a part-time basis. It is not clear how female doctors will take decisions in relation to the new higher scale of investment and managerial commitment required by the new larger general practice 'partnerships'.

6. *Membership of professional organisations* There were some differences in membership of the BMA between areas (Table 4.6). But variations in membership of the RCGP were more clearly related to practice strategy. Innovator practices were much more likely to have at least one partner who was an RCGP member, and among such practices, membership was particularly high in less affluent areas (Tables 4.6 and 5.10). Thus, 47 per cent of innovator practices in the London Inner City area, 63 per cent of such practices in the North East Industrial area and 39 per cent in the North Mining area had at least one partner who was a member of the College. Innovation was significantly related to RCGP membership especially in less affluent areas. There are still questions about causation and it is not clear whether innovation led to RCGP membership or vice versa. But for the present, the partners' professional networks appeared to be important, especially in areas where the economic returns to innovation were lowest.

7. *The payment system* A uniform national payments system has led to considerable variations in gross and net income between areas. Between areas the differences were such that net incomes at the lower quartile in the Thames Valley (£24,200) and East Rural (£30,000) areas were greater than the median value (£23,000) in the Midlands Urban area.The clearest incentive from the payment system was towards increasing partnership size. The costs of larger practices were lower, so that small

differences in gross income between practices of different sizes became much larger differences in net income. Thus the costs of the two partner practices were 46 per cent of gross income and their net income £21,800 per partner. The costs of the 23 five partner practices in the study were 33 per cent of gross income and their net income per partner £27,700 (Table 6.3). The payment system gives clear signals on partnership size up to a partnership size of six. After that, problems of organisation seemed to lead to lower net income. The payment system also gives little incentive to high list size, and even in areas of expanding population, practices were keeping list size per partner to around 2000, any extra patients being accommodated by increasing partnership size.

8. *The local environment* This had strong and complex effects on practices. In some areas it led to a different age structure among family doctors, but the most important effects were on practice size and on practice strategy. Large practices were more common in affluent areas and such practices were more likely to be innovators. However innovation was not just a function of size. Smaller practices were more likely to be innovators in affluent areas than smaller practices elsewhere. The range of area differences in practice strategy was such that 68 per cent of practices in the East Rural area were innovators compared to 23 per cent in the Midlands Urban area.

9. *Practice strategies* Various features of practice staffing and organisation are sometimes described as if they reflected discrete and independent decisions. The concept of 'practice strategy' has been used in this study to examine practice decision-making. A strategy involves a co-ordinated series of decisions on the most important issues facing the practice. The survey evidence does suggest that a number of decisions are linked. As well as taking part in the vocational training scheme (72 per cent), employing a practice nurse (92 per cent) and taking part in the cost rent scheme (72 per cent) which were used to define these practices, innovators were also more likely to employ a practice manager (Table 5.12), and to have a computer within the practice (Table 5.13) than were other types of practices.

Decisions on strategy seemed to be determined mainly by local environment rather than by the personal characteristics of the doctors. Innovator practices were much more likely to have experienced a rise in population in the area around the practice (Table 5.4). The effect can be illustrated from two areas, NW Suburban and Midlands Urban. In the generally affluent NW Suburban area, the innovation rate was high and 58 per cent of innovators had experienced a rise in their local population compared to 37 per cent of traditionalists. In the Midlands Urban area, 46 per cent of the smaller number of innovator practices had experienced a population rise compared to 5 per cent of traditionalist practices. The most striking example of the effects of population change and of local social environment was to be found within the Thames Valley area. In the urban section of the Thames Valley area there were no innovators among nine practices, while in the more suburban and affluent section, 48 per cent of practices - 11 out of 23 - were innovators.

The general practice system aims to encourage investment and change. The Family Doctor Charter has worked well in the more affluent and suburban areas, but the problem of incentives to development and change in a wide range of industrial areas remains.

10. *List size* There were small differences in list size between practices with different strategies or in different areas, but these had significant effects on net income. The reduction of average list size from its current level of approximately 2000 to 1700 has long been a professional target (British Medical Association, 1984). Although this has never been formally accepted as a goal by government, the steady increase in numbers of doctors entering general practice is likely to bring it about within ten years. A detailed study of the effects of list size on practice activity has already thrown some doubt on the benefits of any such policy (Butler and Calnan, 1987) and the current survey raises more questions still. A reduction in average list size to 1700 will mean that larger numbers of practices have very low list sizes. These small practices are the ones which are least likely to innovate and to develop preventive care. A reduction in average list size aimed at improving quality of care may, in fact, make it more difficult for practices to improve quality of care in those areas where it is least likely to be acceptable.

Policies for increasing the number of doctors not only affect list size, they also affect costs both directly, in their effects on pay, and indirectly through the effects on prescriptions and referrals. The increase in numbers of general practitioners also reduces incentives to delegation and to teamwork.

An alternative to the policy of reducing list size would be to stabilise it at around current levels and to encourage joint working with practices locally to enhance viability. The change would affect levels of medical manpower and would increase the case for a re-assessment of levels of entry to medical schools. The higher productivity of larger general practices is likely to mean that general practice cannot absorb new manpower as it has done in the past. Britain has been one of the last countries not to have a surplus of doctors, but current policies for increasing numbers in general practice seem likely to create such a surplus. Policies for practice development at the local level need to be accompanied by a re-assessment of policies for medical manpower at the national level.

11. *Partnership size* Differences in partnership size are closely related to strategies and outcomes. Larger practices were more likely to be innovators. 19 per cent of two partner practices were innovators compared to 44 per cent of those with four partners and 72 per cent of five partner practices (Table 5.16). Larger practices had higher average net incomes and lower costs. Average net income for two partner practices was £21,800 as compared to £27,700 for five partner practices (Table 6.3). Larger practices serve many more patients. Differences in list size per partner may have been equalised but differences in practice size have become more significant.

12. *Outcomes for doctors* Local environment conditions practice strategy, and in turn shapes outcomes. The returns to innovation are favourable in the more affluent areas but not elsewhere. The effect of innovation in the less affluent areas is to raise income above the area average but to leave them below the national average. Thus the net income of innovators in the Midlands Urban area was £25,000 and in the North Mining Area £25,400, compared to £27,300 for all practices. Such figures have to be seen against a background of much higher consultation rates for practices in less affluent areas. On a regional basis, consultation rates varied in 1986 from 3.1 consultations per head of population in East Anglia to 4.9 per head in the North West (Office of Health Economics, 1987).

The system works to reward innovation in the more affluent areas and to provide a poor return elsewhere. The pattern of capital investment points to the same conclusion. Innovators had invested in their premises more heavily in all areas, and the level of investment in the less affluent areas was much the same as in areas where property prices were likely to rise quickly to cover the investment (Table 6.11). Thus the degree of personal risk taken by innovators in the less affluent areas in undertaking investments greater than the current market value of the property was much greater.

13. *Services for patients* The survey evidence showed that innovator and intermediate practices were more likely than traditionalists to have had special clinics for many years (Table 7.1). In addition, innovator practices were more likely than others to have an appointment system (Table 7.6) and an age/sex register (Table 7.7) which suggests a higher degree of practice organisation, perhaps also linked to the larger average partnership size of innovator practices. Innovator practices, being larger, were also more likely to have branch surgeries.

14. *The hypotheses* The first chapter set out three initial hypotheses about practice strategy. Practice strategy would be influenced by the professional and personal characteristics of the doctors and it would also be conditioned by the local environment. Decisions on practice strategy would, in turn, have certain financial outcomes so that practices which were most active in developing services would face the greatest financial pressure.

In terms of personal characteristics the clearest effect seemed to be from membership of professional organisations, especially in less affluent areas. The professional networks to which a doctor is related seemed to influence decisions on practice strategy. Differences in professional contacts and motivation were also reflected in the considerable area differences in participation in the vocational training scheme. Thus 49 per cent of practices in Area 1 (NW Suburban), had at least one partner who was a trainer compared to 19 per cent of practices in the Midlands Urban area (Table 4.16). Ethnic background also seemed to have important effects.

The strongest effect on practice strategy seemed to be from the local environment. Practices in areas of expanding population were much more likely to be innovators. The effect was important within, as well as between, areas. 44 per cent of innovators had experienced a population rise in their local environment compared to 16 per cent of traditionalists (Table 5.4). The area effect seemed to work partly through larger partnership size, so that large partnerships were more likely to be found in the more affluent areas. However, small practices were also more likely to be innovators in the more affluent areas.

The results from the third hypothesis were mixed. The returns to innovation were clear in the more affluent areas, and innovation seemed to be a guarantee against a low income defined in terms of a net income of less than £20,000 a year. But in less affluent areas, innovator practices had higher costs and the incentives to innovation appeared to be weak.

Policy development

The Family Doctor Charter (British Medical Association, 1965) favoured teamwork in general practice. There were no cash limits nor financial constraints on development, but there were incentives to improve premises, to take on extra staff, and to adopt larger partnerships. Policies influencing professional aspirations were less common. The most important was the vocational training scheme, but there were no policies to influence retirement or the age distribution of family doctors.

It has often been predicted that family doctors could take over functions of the hospital (British Medical Association, 1984). It may well be that technology is now changing in ways that will make this a reality.

> "Analytical procedures, previously only able to be performed in custom built laboratories staffed by highly-trained technicians and scientists, can now be carried out by relatively unskilled personnel in the clinic or on the ward without loss of precision or accuracy" (Marks, 1985).

> "Near patient testing is an everyday reality which has come about largely as a result of developments in the electronics, computer or diagnostic reagents industries. These developments have led to construction of simple micro-processor controlled instruments that can be used in conjunction with various types of physico-chemical sensors to produce reliable and accurate quantitative data.... With such instrumentation virtually anyone... can obtain an analytical result with acceptable precision and accuracy within minutes of sample collection at an overall cost no greater and possibly less, than if it had been transported to a laboratory" (Marks, 1985a).

Any new policy framework will have to provide opportunities for investment in working capital. The White Paper (Department of Health and Social Security, 1987) set out a regime with the following main features.

(a) A professional model providing preventive, effective and accessible care.

(b) An economic regime to achieve the aim of competition.

"No opportunity should be lost to increase fair and open competition between those providing Family Practitioner Services" (Department of Health and Social Security, 1987). Competition, it is alleged, will stimulate doctors to increase the range and quality of services which they provide.

(c) Financial incentives which link pay to performance and to the range of services provided. The incentives could include an increased role for capitation fees, so that the fees would rise to 50 per cent of total remuneration from their current level of 48 per cent. In addition there would be new fees for meeting immunisation targets, for check ups on patients registering with the National Health Service for the first time, for providing full care for elderly patients, and for monitoring child development.

(d) Family Practitioner Committees and family doctors are to work together to achieve certain local targets, such as a certain level of immunisation uptake which will differ depending on the current level of such services within an area. To provide additional services, it might be necessary for practices to improve or extend their premises, employ a wider range of ancillary staff and take on more partners. The

White Paper has added this management role to the planning role given to Family Practitioners Committees in 1984 (Allsop and May, 1986).

(e) An aspiration that the health care 'consumer' will be prepared to 'shop around' for a wider variety of medical service being offered by practices.

If implemented, the effects of these incentives and management initiatives cannot be seen in isolation from other policies at national level. Policy on average list size will affect the ability of practices to add to income through increased capitation fees. Decisions about future levels of medical manpower will affect the numbers of doctors seeking to enter general practice. It may become easier for larger practices to employ part-time staff as numbers of female doctors increase. If single handed practitioners continue to crowd into inner city areas this will have the effect of reducing returns to innovation in such areas.

What are the main implications from the survey and from the past record in policy making, about this approach in the White Paper? General practice is likely to be involved in another period of change which will have fundamental effects. The survey results can give some assistance in assessing the various elements in the structure. The key themes which emerge are:

The likely area differences in the impact of fees for service

The survey results have implications for the financial incentives advocated in the White Paper, in which fees were suggested for providing check-up examinations for patients new to the National Health Service, for paediatric surveillance, and for regular care of the elderly. Innovator practices in affluent areas are in a much stronger position to increase their income from such fees. They face a heavier demand for their services, are under less pressure from a high rate of consultations, and are better able to organise the call and recall and information systems that are required to increase income from such fees, especially as the results showed that they were more likely to have computers. A swing towards more fee for service is likely to mean a further widening of the differences in net income between practices in the affluent areas and elsewhere.

The obstacles facing practices not just in inner cities, but more widely

The survey results did not support the assumption of the White Paper on primary care that special problems of development are concentrated in a few inner city areas (Department of Health and Social Security, 1987). The incentives for practices to innovate have had a weak impact throughout industrial areas. Even within the classification 'inner cities' there are distinct differences between inner London and the Manchester-Salford area (Wood, 1983). The study results further strengthen the case for using a term such as 'area of developmental difficulty' rather than inner city, and for applying more explicit criteria for choosing such areas. Such criteria might cover variables of need, such as indicators of social deprivation, and also variables of supply, such as the structure of practices and the degree of response to innovation within an area. Unless help in terms of management and resources is given to practices in such areas, it seems unlikely that they will show greater responses to the new incentives than they did to the old ones.

The White Paper (Department of Health and Social Security, 1987) advocated the extension of fee for service, but did not consider the possible impact of these proposals on practice organisation. The evidence of area variability from the survey suggests that the management role is going to be critical. The aim of "better" primary care will vary in feasibility with social conditions and demography. The service priorities will be very different in different areas. The problems of developing new services will depend on practice strategy. The complexity of the changes required also means that the payment of fees for service may not be a very effective way of getting them. For example, it is hoped that family doctors will provide "comprehensive regular care for elderly people" (Department of Health and Social Security, 1987). This would take time, teamwork, and the information and motivation required to give effective support to frail elderly people.

The new role of the Family Practitioner Committees will involve them in more active management of primary care and there will be more awareness of the scale of the duplication and possible competition between out-patient services, the family doctor service and community nursing. The White Paper may want to see an expansion of primary care, but locally this will only make sense if there is less duplication with the school health service and with hospital out-patient departments, and this will only happen if there is a shared management approach between Family Practitioner Committee and District Health Authorities.

A new approach to expansion of primary care through a local programme budget or primary care fund would be one possibility (Bosanquet, 1986). Funding should be related to local plans for developing primary care. Costs could be identified separately from income so as to assist practices with start-up costs. Programme finance would make it much easier to link decisions by practices on their strategies, to local definitions of need.

The White Paper recommended that Family Practitioner Committees should get involved in supply side planning but it did not do enough to make use of an unusual opportunity to attract new recruits, or to improve practice structure in the older industrial areas as well as in the inner city. Concern with planning in primary care has had its main focus on the demand side and on the measurement of need but there is a great deal of scope for active supply side planning. The survey results show that the response to incentives by practices could be quite strong. Supply side planning would allow full use to be made of this potential in the future.

The first requirement is for the development of an information base about current and prospective changes in practices. Information on change in age structure is relevant. It is also essential to have information on changes in income, costs and list size, which might affect the viability of practices. The local results suggest connections running from practice structure through to service availability. Family Practitioner Committees are in a position to collect data which will give some guide to the viability of practices.

The information could be used to develop new kinds of policies, if additional management resources were available to do this. Such policies cannot guarantee innovation and service development but they can create conditions in which it is more likely to happen. Some examples of policies recommended in an area where these methods were applied are as follows (Bosanquet, 1987).

(1) To offer existing practices the option of expansion in an area by taking on extra partners when single-handed practitioners retire. The first priority should be to strengthen existing practices with development potential.

(2) To group single handed vacancies when they occur and to offer them as partnerships, where none of the existing practices wished to take on extra partners. The Family Practitioner Committee could invite doctors bidding for these practice vacancies to put forward development plans in terms of premises, staffing and services.

(3) To work with existing practices on development plans. These would identify service needs not being met, problems impeding practices in their day to day work and opportunities for collaboration and joint planning. It is difficult to see how Family Practitioner Committees can collaborate with District Health Authorities unless they develop this new kind of relationship with practitioners.

These are examples of policies that were relevant for one Family Practitioner Committee in an inner city, and have been selected as an illustration of the type of approach which has actually been developed by one Family Practitioner Committee. (Bosanquet, 1987) In other areas other policies will be relevant. The general aim of supply side planning is for the Family Practitioner Committee to work with local practices to put the resources available locally to more effective use and to create conditions for practices which will encourage innovation. Such planning is likely to be even more relevant under the conditions created by the government's proposed policies for primary care. Family Practitioner Committees can work with local practices over a period of time to bring about substantial changes in practice structure, which would be essential for the changes in services and in patterns of care advocated in the White Paper to be carried out.

Conclusions

There has been much discussion of various aims and aspirations for improving primary care, and proposals for new incentives. Any system of incentives at the national level will be affected by the forces operating in the local environment. This study has aimed to examine the problems from the doctor's point of view. There are many able and committed people now working in general practice and the potential for better primary care is clearly there.

References

ACARD Report (1986), *Medical Equipment*, London, Department of Health and Social Security.

Alford, R.H. (1975), *Health Care Politics*, Chicago, University of Chicago Press.

Allsop, J. and May, M. (1986), *The Emperor's New Clothes: Family Practitioner Committees in the 1980's*, London, King Edward's Hospital Fund.

Boan, J.A. (1966), *Group Practice*, Ottawa Royal Commission on Health Services, Queens Printer.

Bond, J., Cartlidge, A., Gregson, B., Barton, A., Philips, P., Armitage, P., Brown, A. and Reedy, B. (1987), Interprofessional collaboration in primary health care, *Journal of the Royal College of General Practitioners* 37, 158 -161.

Bosanquet, N. (1986), GPs as firms: creating an internal market for primary care, *Public Money* 5, 45-48.

Bosanquet, N. (1987), *The outlook for General Practice in Kensington and Chelsea and Westminster*, Kensington and Chelsea and Westminster Family Practitioner Committee.

Bosanquet, N. and Leese, B. (1986), Family doctors: Their choice of practice strategy, *British Medical Journal* 293, 667-70.

Bosanquet, N. and Leese, B. (1988), Family doctors and innovation in general practice, *British Medical Journal* 296, 1576 -80.

Bowling, A. (1981), *Delegation in General Practice*, London, Tavistock.

Bradford Hill, A. (1951), The Doctor's pay and day, *Journal of the Royal Statistical Society* CIV, 1-34.

British Medical Association (1965), *A Charter for the Family Doctor Service*, London,

British Medical Association.
British Medical Association (1984), *General Practice: a British Success*, London, General Medical Services Committee.
British Medical Journal (1977), General Practice Premises, *British Medical Journal* 2, 1432.
British Medical Journal (1979), Providing capital for general practice, *British Medical Journal* 1, 1294-5.
British Medical Journal (1981), Valuation of GPs' premises, *British Medical Journal* 282, 1252.
British Medical Journal (1981a), GPFC's new lease back scheme, *British Medical Journal* 282, 1172.
Brown, A.M., Jachuck, S.J., Walters, F., van Zwanenberg, T.D. (1986), The future of general practice in Newcastle upon Tyne, *Lancet* i, 370-371.
Bryan, J. (1986), Treat patients to hi tech medicine in the surgery, *Medeconomics*, September, 33-36.
Butler, J.R. (1980), *How many patients. A study of list sizes in general practice*, Occasional Paper on Social Administration 64, London, Bedford Square Press.
Butler, J.R., Bevan, J.M. and Taylor R.C. (1973), *Family Doctors and Public Policy*, London, Routledge and Kegan Paul.
Butler, J.R. and Calnan, M. (1987), *Too many patients?* London, Gower Publishing Company.
Cabinet Office (1960), *Royal Commission on doctors' and dentists' remuneration 1957-60*, London, HMSO, Cmnd. 939.
Cameron, J. (1983), GP trainees must have passed MRCGP exam, *Pulse* 43, no. 38, 1.
Cartwright, A. (1967), *Patients and their doctors*, London, Routledge.
Cartwright, A. and Anderson, R. (1981), *General Practice Revisited*, London, Tavistock Publications.
Cartwright, A. and Marshall, R. (1965), General Practice in 1963, its conditions, contents and satisfactions, *Medical Care* 3, 69-87.
Chinque, P. (1984), Micros for GPs scheme, *British Journal of Health Care Computing* 1, no. 1, 4-7.
Clayton, G. (1984), Computers in Primary Care, *British Journal of Health Care Computing* 1, no. 1, 18-22.
Cochrane, A. (1973), *Effectiveness and efficiency. Some random reflections on health services*, London, Nuffield Provincial Hospitals Trust.
Collings, J.S. (1950), General Practice in England Today; a reconnaissance, *Lancet* i, 555-585.
Cullis, J. and West, P. (1979), *The Economics of Health. An Introduction*, Oxford, Martin Robertson.
Davidson, J. (1982), The practice nurse grows up, *Nursing Mirror* 154, no. 3, ii-iv.
Denham, C. (1984), Urban Britain, *Population Trends* 36, 10-18.
Department of Employment (1986), Self-employment in Britain, *Employment Gazette* vol. 94, no. 5, 183-194.
Department of Health and Social Security (1981), Acheson Report. London Health Planning Consortium Primary Health Care Study Group, *Primary Health Care in Inner London*, London, Department of Health and Social Security.

Department of Health and Social Security (1984), *Evaluation of the micros for GPs*

scheme. Interim Report, London, HMSO.
Department of Health and Social Security (1985), *Evaluating the micros for GPs scheme. Final report*, London, HMSO.
Department of Health and Social Security (1986), *Primary Health Care; an Agenda for discussion*, London, HMSO, Cmnd. 9777.
Department of Health and Social Security, (1986a), *Neighbourhood Nursing - A Focus for Care*, Report of the Community Nursing Review, London, HMSO.
Department of Health and Social Security (1986b), *General Practice Finance Corporation*, Press Release, 9.7.86.
Department of Health and Social Security (1986c), *Micros in Practice*, Report of an appraisal of GP microcomputer systems, London, HMSO.
Department of Health and Social Security (1986d), *A prescription for change*, A report on the longer term use and development of computers in general practice, London, HMSO.
Department of Health and Social Security (1987), *Promoting Better Health*, London, HMSO, Cmnd. 249.
Department of Health and Social Security (1987a), *Health and Personal Social Services Statistics for England*, London, HMSO.
Department of Health and Social Security (1987b), *General medical practitioners' workload*, A report prepared for the Doctors' and Dentists' Review Body, 1985/86, Department of Health and Social Security.
Digby, A. and Bosanquet, N. (1988), Doctors and Patients in an era of National Health insurance and private practice, *Economic History Review* XLI, 1, 74-94.
Dowie, R. (1983), *General Practitioners and Consultants*, London, King Edward's Hospital Fund.
Enthoven, A. (1985), *Reflections on the management of the National Health Service*, London, Nuffield Provincial Hospital Trust.
Feldstein, M. (1970), The rising price of physicians' services, *The Review of Economics and Statistics*, L11, no. 2, 121-133.
Fowler, G. (1986), Prevention, in Fry, J. and Hasler, J., *Primary Health Care 2000*, London, Churchill Livingstone.
Fox, J. (1984), *Linear statistical models and related methods*, London, Wiley.
Fisher, R.H. (1984), A complete system for the family practitioner service, *British Journal of Health Care Computing*, 1 no. 4, 10-12.
Fry, J. (1986), *Journal of the Royal College of General Practitioners' Members' Reference Book*, London, RCGP.
Fry, J. and Hasler, J. (1986), *Primary Health Care 2000*, London, Churchill Livingstone.
General Practice Finance Corporation (1986), *Annual Report*, London, House of Commons 526.
General Practitioner (1982), Dawn of a new age for GPs, *General Practitioner* 13 August 1982, 13.
Hall, D. (1986), Try a surgery conversion , *Medeconomics* March, 88-90.
Ham, C. (1981), *Policy making in the National Health Service*, London, Macmillan.
Hansard (1982), *General Practitioner (Computers)* no. 1247, 11-17th June.
Hansard (1983), *Family Doctors (Inner Cities)*, no. 1249, 14-18th December.
Harker, P. Leopoldt, H. and Robinson, J.R. (1976), Attaching community psychiat-

ric nurses to general practice, *Journal of the Royal College of General Practitioners* 20, 6-12.
Hart, J.T. (1985), Practice nurses, an underused resource, *British Medical Journal* 290, 1162.
Hay, J., Acheson R.M., Reiss B.B., Evans, C.E. (1980), Teachers in general practice: a comparative study, *Medical Education* 14, 277-254.
Honigsbaum, F. (1979), *The Division in British Medicine*, London, Kogan Page.
Horder, J., Bosanquet, N. and Stocking, B. (1986), Ways of influencing the behaviour of general practitioners, *Journal of the Royal College of General practitioners* 36, no.2, 517-521.
House of Commons Social Services Committee (1987), *Public expenditure on the social services*, memorandum from the DHSS, London, HMSO.
Hunter, D.J. (1980), *Coping with uncertainty. Policy and politics in the National Health Service*, Research Studies Press.
Irvine, D. and Jeffreys, M. (1971), BMA planning unit survey of general practice 1969, *British Medical Journal* 4, 535-543.
Jessop, M. (1984), Why some doctors seem to like their chips, *General Practitioner* 4th May, 22.
Joint Committee on Postgraduate Training for General Practice (1980), *Criteria for selection of trainees in general practice*, London, JCPTGP.
Josse, E. (1981), Using the ECG in general practice, *Pulse* 41, 39.
Jowell, R. and Airey, C. (1984), *British Social Attitudes. The 1984 Report*, London, Gower.
Kuenssberg, E.V. (1980), The impact of technology on general practice, *Journal of Medical Engineering Technology* 4, 170-171.
Kurji, K.H. and Haines, A.P. (1984), Detection and management of hypertension in general practice, *British Medical Journal* 288, 903-906.
Lancet (1984), Towards better general practice, *The Lancet* ii, 1436-8.
Lowe, M. (1981), Premises pay for GPs, *Medeconomics*, August, 6.
Lowe, M. (1981a), Modernise your surgeries with FPC cash, *Medeconomics*, December, 16.
Lowe, M. (1982), Staff wage repayment, *Medeconomics*, February, 16.
Lowe, M. (1982a), Check you get the best in rent and rates, *Medeconomics*, January, 14.
Lyall, J. (1979), Consider the importance of counsellors in practice, *General Practitioner*, 3rd August, 7-8.
Mair, A. and Mair, G.B. (1959), Five year study of a general practice, *British Medical Journal supplement*, 20th June, 281-284.
Marks, V. (1985), The trend towards decentralisation, lessons from history, in Marks, V. and Alberti, K. (eds), *Clinical Biochemistry Nearer the patient*, Edinburgh, Churchill Livingstone.
Marks, V. (1985a), Near-patient testing - an overview, in Marks, V. and Alberti, K. (eds), *Clinical Biochemistry Nearer the Patient*, Edinburgh, Churchill Livingstone.
Marsh, G. and Kaim-Caudle, P. (1976), *Team Care in General Practice*, London, Croom Helm.
Marsh, G. and McNay, R.A. (1974), Team workload in an English general practice, *British Medical Journal* 1, 315-318.
Marsh, G. (1982), Are follow-up consultations at medical out-patient departments futile? *British Medical Journal* 284, 1176-1177.

McKeown, T. (1979), *The role of Medicine* , Oxford, Basil Blackwell.
Medical Services Review Committee (1962), *A Review of the Medical Services in Great Britain*, London, Social Assay.
Metcalfe, D., Wilkin, D., Hodgkin, P., Hallam, L., Cooke, M. (1983), *A study of the process of care in urban general practice.*, University of Manchester, Department of Health and Social Security. Primary Care Research Unit.
Michael, G. (1981), New medical equipment for the practice, *Pulse* 14, 62-63.
Ministry of Health and Department of Health for Scotland 'Spens' Report (1946), *Committee on the remuneration of General Practitioners*, London, HMSO, Cmnd. 6810.
Ministry of Health (1968), *The field of work of the Family doctor*, London, HMSO.
Morrison, D.E. andHenkel, R.E. (1970), *The significance test controversy*, London, Heinemann.
NAHA (1988), *New horizons in acute care*, King Edward's Hospital Fund for London.
National Audit Office (1988), *Management of the family practitioner services*, London, HMSO.
Nenk, B. (1982), Regional coordinators get free computers, *Pulse* 42, 2.
OECD (1987), *Financing and Delivering Health Care: a Comparative Analysis of OECD Countries*, Paris, OECD.
Office of Health Economics (1987), *Compendium of Health Statistics.*
OPCS (1983), *Census 1981* Great Britain, HMSO.
Palmer, P. and Rees, C. (1980), *Computing in General Practice*, A report for the GMSC of the BMA, London, Scicon Consultancy International.
Pauly, M. (1980), *Doctors and their workshops. Economic models of physician behaviour*, Chicago, University of Chicago Press.
Pettigrew, A. (1985), *The awakening giant. Continuity and change in ICI*, Blackwell.
Pike, L.A., Beaumont, C.D. and Clewett, A.J. (1981), *Morbidity and environment in an urban general practice*, London, HMSO.
Reedy, B.L.E.C., Burton, A.G., Gregson, B.A., Brown, A.M., Cartlidge, A.M.,Stanley, J., Bolam, F., Bond, J. and Russell, I.T. (1983), *Professional collaboration in primary care*, University of Newcastle upon Tyne, Health Care Research Unit, Report No. 24.
Rees, A.J. and Shultz, G.P. (1970), *Workers and wages in an urban labour market*, Chicago, University of ChicagoPress.
Reinhardt, U. (1972), A production function for physician services, *Review of Economics and Statistics* 53, no.l, 55-66.
Review Body on Doctors' and Dentists' Remuneration (1987), *Seventeenth Report*, London, HMSO, Cmnd. 127.
Ritchie, L.D. (1982), Computers in general practice: a review of the current situation, *Health Bulletin*, 40, 248-254.
Ross, J.D. (1952), *The National Health Service in Great Britain*, OUP, (includes full text of Danckwerts' award).
Routh, G. (1980), *Occupation and pay in Great Britain 1906-79*, London, Macmillan.
Royal College of General Practitioners (1980), *Computers in Primary Care*, Interim report, London, RCGP.
Royal College of General Practitioners (1980a), *Hypertension in Primary Care*, Occasional paper no.12, London, RCGP.

Royal College of General Practitioners, (1981), *The measurement of the quality of General Practitioner Care*, Occasional paper no. 15, London, RCGP.

Royal College of General Practitioners (1981a), A *survey of primary care in London*, Occasional paper no. 16, London, RCGP.

Royal College of General Practitioners (1982), *Computers in Primary Care*, Report of the Computer Working Party, Occasional paper no.13, London, RCGP.

Royal College of General Practitioners (1982a), *Inner Cities*, Occasional paper no. 19, London, RCGP.

Royal College of General Practitioners (1982b), *Medical Audit in General Practice*, Occasional paper no. 20, London, RCGP.

Royal College of General Practitioners (1982c), *The influence of trainers on trainees in General Practice*, Occasional paper no. 21, London, RCGP.

Royal College of General Practitioners (1985), *Towards quality in General Practice*, London, RCGP.

Royal College of General Practitioners (1985a), *What sort of doctor*, London, RCGP.

Russell, W. (1981), Government and Opposition in harmony on GPFC, *British Medical Journal* 282, 1808.

Siddy, K. (1987), Why many big partnerships have cut back their numbers, *Medeconomics* 8, No. 3, 54-58.

Steen, P. (1967), Some aspects of group practice, *The Practitioner* 199, 810-813.

Stoddart, N. (1984), Computers in perspective, *Practice Computing* 3, no. 1, 16-17.

Stoddart, N. (1985), A little light evaluation, *Practice Computing* 4, no. 1, 16-17.

Wilkin, D., Hallam, L., Leavey, R., Metcalfe, D. (1987), *Anatomy of urban General Practice*, London, Tavistock.

Williams, P. and Clare, A. (1979), Social Workers in primary health care: the general practitioner's viewpoint, *Journal of the Royal College of General Practitioners* 29, 554-558.

Wood, J. (1983), Are the Problems of Primary Health care in inner cities fact or fiction? *British Medical Journal* 286, 1109-1112.

Woodward, R.S. and Warren Boulton, F. (1984), Considering the effects of financial incentives and professional ethics on appropriate medical care, *Journal of Health Economics*, vol. 3, no. 3, 223-237.

World Health Organisation (1978), *Primary Health Care*, Geneva, WHO/UNICEF.

Appendix 1
A statistical analysis

In addition to tabulation and selective graphical displays, the statistical relationships between innovators and various potential explanatory factors has been explored by using regression methods. In particular a body of technique known as *logit modelling* which takes account of the categorical nature of much of the information available was used.

The usual techniques of regression begin with a dependent variable which can take *any* value (albeit that some values will occur only with small probabilities) and seek to account for the variation which this exhibits by means of one or more explanatory variables which determine the 'systematic component' of the regression model. The starting point in this study is a dependent variable with two values ('innovator' and 'other'), coded for the purposes of the analysis as either 0 or 1. The word 'logit' refers to a mathematical transformation which overcomes the difficulty caused by the dichotomous nature of the dependent variable (Fox, 1984).

These techniques produce approximate tests of statistical significance. The reservations which have been expressed concerning the use of significance tests in social research (Morrison and Henkel, 1970) are well known. Nevertheless, statistical tests do provide a means by which the magnitude of differences and effects may be judged and it is with this in mind that these results have been reported, leaving it to the reader to add any further reservations which she or he feels are necessary.

The potential explanatory variables themselves are also best considered as 'factors' (with categorical 'levels') rather than as variables with numerical values. Whether or not the practice had an Asian or a female partner are obvious instances of two level factors; such quantities as 'partnership size' and 'average age', although measured on a numerical scale, were redefined to three levels. A full definition of the factors used is given below. There are a large number of possible ways of specifying the systematic component of the model and the results reported here were selected partly by reference to prior hypotheses and partly from preliminary data analysis. This is, of course, one reason for treating tests of statistical significance with caution. Not all possible 'models' could be investigated and not all results are reported here.

The first step in the exploration was to remove all cases which fell into the 'intermediate' class of practices, leaving 150 cases who are either 'traditionalist' or 'innovator'. Of these, 10 cases were unusable because information on practice income was not available. The factors considered are as follows:

Name	*Definition*
RCGP membership	whether at least one partner is a member of the RCGP Level 1: no RCGP members in the practice Level 2: at least one partner is RCGP member
Average net income	average net income per head (not fte) Level 1: < 15,000 Level 2: 15,001 - 20,000 Level 3: 20,001 - 25,000 Level 4: 25,001 - 30,000 Level 5: 30,001 - 40,000 Level 6: > 40,001
Partnership size	Level 1: 2 or 3 partners in practice Level 2: 4 or 5 partners in practice Level 3: more than 5 partners
Asian partner	whether or not the partnership has at least one Asian partner Level 1: no Asian partners in practice Level 2: at least one partner is Asian
Health centre	whether or not the partnership operates from a health centre Level 1: Practice does not operate from a health centre Level 2: Practice operates from a health centre
Female doctor	whether or not the partnership has at least one female partner Level 1: no female partners in practice Level 2: at least one partner is female
Average age	average age of the partnership Level 1: < 40 years Level 2: 40 - 50 years Level 3: > 50 years
Area	area in which the partnership is situated Level 1: Less affluent areas - London Inner City, North East Industrial, Midlands Urban Level 2: More affluent areas - NW Suburban, Thames Valley, East Rural

For the benefit of readers who are unacquainted with the techniques of analysis used here, four preliminary points can be made to assist interpretation. Firstly, it will be seen that the 'model' is defined by a set of 'coefficients' (the numbers printed under the heading 'estimate' in the sections which follow); one coefficient is identified by the word 'Constant' and the others associated with each of the factor levels beyond the first. Where the explanatory power of just one factor is reported, this means that the constant is associated with the 'lowest' level of the factor and the succeeding coefficients quantify the (average) effect on the dependent variable at the second, third ... factor levels. Where the use of two or more factors is explored, the 'constant' represents the combined effect of all the factors at their lowest levels.

The second point is to observe that the 'effect' of factors may be thought of as altering the estimated *probability* that a practice is an innovator. Thus, a positive coefficient suggests that the probability is increased by the presence of that factor level in a practice; a negative coefficient has the effect of lowering the probability.

It may help to illustrate these last two points - and explain the term 'logit' - by means of a simple example. Taking the results relating to the joint effect of 'Asian partner' and 'Area' we have:

	estimate	s.e.	t
Constant	0.504	0.305	1.65
Asian partner	-1.471	0.457	-3.22
Area	0.672	0.392	1.71

As noted above, the constant refers to the two 'factors' - Asian partner and Area - at their lowest levels, which are 'no Asian partner' and 'less affluent area'. The figure 0.504 is mathematically the logarithm of the estimated odd that a practice is innovative and is called the *logit*, notationally:

$$\log\left(\frac{p}{1-p}\right)$$

where p denotes the estimated probability that the practice is innovative. The logarithms are natural logarithms and hence:

$$\exp(0.504) = 1.65 = p/(1-p)$$

from which, by simple rearrangement, p is found to be 0.62. When one of the other factors - say Asian partner - is at its second level (one or more Asian partners), the logit becomes

$$0.504 - 1.471 = -0.967$$

and therefore p/(1-p) is 0.38, giving a value for p of 0.28. In this way do negative and positive 'effects' - as quantified by the reported coefficients - determine the estimated probability that a practice exhibiting a particular configuration of factors levels is innovative.

The third point concerns the quantity described as the 'deviance'. The *total* deviance may be thought of as a measure of the 'variability' of the dependent variable across the data. As the dependent variable remains the 'innovator/non innovator' split throughout the investigation, the total deviance also remains as 186.7. Mathematically, it can be shown that this 'total' deviance can be broken down into two components, namely a component 'explained' by the factor (or factors) - this is the entry in the row labelled 'Regression' in the analysis of deviance table - and a 'Residual' deviance. Each 'deviance' has a certain number of 'degrees of freedom' associated with it; these are shown in the column headed 'd.f.' The *total* degrees of freedom are calculated as the number of cases available for analysis - 1, in this case 139; the 'regression' degrees of freedom are equal to the number of coefficients *not counting the constant term*. A test of the significance of a relationship (at the conventional 5 per cent level) may be made by comparing the 'regression' deviance with the 0.05 probability value in a table of the χ^2 distribution: a 'large' regression deviance typically being significant. The significance of factor levels may be judged by examination of the entries in the columns headed 's.e.' (standard error). In general, a t-ratio whose value is greater than 2 (ignoring the sign) suggests that the corresponding factor level is significantly different from the 'base' level (the constant term).

The final point concerns the consequences of using two or more factors to explain the variation in innovation levels. Taken together, factors effects are not (usually) additive, that is to say that the effect of, say, partnership size and the presence/absence of an Asian partner together *cannot* be deduced by considering the effects separately. A similar problem is often observed in more conventional regression.

Finally, two further general points on the exploration of these data may be made. The first is that an alternative analysis not reported here has been conducted with 'innovators' defined as 'innovators' (as here) plus 'intermediates' with broadly similar conclusions to those shown in the following sections. Secondly, the decision to work with 'area' as defined above was made after inspection of results based upon area defined at the six levels which have been used in the main body of this book; again, the conclusions are similar to those reported here. (Area 7 is excluded from the analysis). The statistical calculations were made with the computing system Genstat (Mark 5). The results follow.

Relationships between practice characteristics and the innovation decision

1 *Presence/absence of Asian partner(s)*

	estimate	s.e.	t
Constant	0.897	0.213	4.22
Asian partner	-1.730	0.433	-3.99

ANALYSIS OF DEVIANCE

	d.f.	deviance
Regression	1	17.4
Residual	138	169.3
Total	139	186.7

Comment: The presence of at least one Asian partner has a statistically significant negative association with innovation (the critical value of χ^2 at the 5% level is 3.84).

2 *Presence/absence of female partner(s)*

	estimate	s.e.	t
Constant	0.236	0.244	0.97
Female partner	0.457	0.349	1.31

ANALYSIS OF DEVIANCE

	d.f.	deviance
Regression	1	1.7
Residual	138	185.0
Total	139	186.7

Comment: The presence of a female partner has no statistically significant effect on the innovation decision (the critical value of χ^2 at the 5% level is 3.84).

3 *Effect of age*

	estimate	s.e.	t
Constant	0.511	0.326	1.57
Average age (level 2)	0.182	0.395	0.46
Average age (level 3)	-2.71	1.10	-2.45

ANALYSIS OF DEVIANCE

	d.f.	deviance
Regression	2	12.7
Residual	137	174.0
Total	139	186.7

Comment: The average age of the partnership has a statistically significant negative effect at its highest level on the innovation decision (the critical value of χ^2 at the 5% level is 5.99).

4 *Effect of working from a health centre*

	estimate	s.e.	t
Constant	0.000	0.316	0.00
Practice in a health centre	0.663	0.380	1.75

ANALYSIS OF DEVIANCE

	d.f.	deviance
Regression	1	3.0
Residual	138	183.7
Total	139	186.7

Comment: The effect of working from a health centre makes no statistically significant reduction in the deviance (the critical value of χ^2 at the 5% level is 3.84).

5 *The effect of one or more partners being members of the RCGP*

	estimate	s.e.	t
Constant	-0.279	0.250	-1.11
RCGP membership	1.506	0.372	4.04

ANALYSIS OF DEVIANCE

	d.f.	deviance
Regression	1	17.6
Residual	138	169.1
Total	139	186.7

Comment: Membership of the RCGP makes a statistically significant reduction in deviance (the critical value of χ^2 at the 5% level is 3.84).

6 *Effect of average net income*

		estimate	s.e.	t
Constant		-1.012	0.582	-1.74
Average net income	level 2	0.845	0.712	1.19
	level 3	1.508	0.673	2.24
	level 4	1.481	0.707	2.09
	level 5	2.621	0.760	3.45
	level 6	2.96	1.21	2.45

ANALYSIS OF DEVIANCE

	d.f.	deviance
Regression	5	19.4
Residual	134	167.3
Total	139	186.7

Comment: Increasing average net income is positively associated with the decision to innovate (the critical value of χ^2 at the 5% level is 11.07).

7 *Effect of partnership size*

	estimate	s.e.	t
Constant	-0.427	0.235	-1.82
Partnership size 4 - 5 partners	2.373	0.527	4.50
Partnership size > 5 partners	2.373	0.653	3.63

ANALYSIS OF DEVIANCE

	d.f.	deviance
Regression	2	36.5
Residual	137	150.2
Total	139	186.7

Comment: There is an increasing and statistically significant association between partnership size and the innovation decision (the critical value of χ^2 at the 5% level is 5.99).

The results of a stepwise regression approach

Using a stepwise approach, the following appears as the most satisfactory set of factors to explain the innovation decision (no further term added was statistically significant):

	estimate	s.e.	t
Constant	0.234	0.396	0.592
Partnership size 4 - 5 partners	2.088	0.552	3.78
Partnership size > 5 partners	1.934	0.681	2.84
Asian partner	-1.563	0.493	-3.17
Average age (level 2)	-0.019	0.463	-0.04
Average age (level 3)	-2.14	1.13	-1.89

with summary analysis of deviance as follows:

	d.f.	deviance
Regression	5	52.2
Residual	134	134.5
Total	139	186.7

The components of deviance are as follows:

	d.f.	deviance
Partnership size	2	36.511
Asian partner	1	10.042
Average age	2	5.603
Residual	134	134.547
Total	139	186.702

Comments: All factors contribute statistically significant reductions to the deviance at the 5% level or better. The positive effects of larger partnership size and the negative effects of Asian partnership and being in an older average age band are apparent. The critical values of χ^2 (at the 5% level) are: 1 df 3.84; 2 df 5.99; 5 df 11.07.

The effects of area (at 2 levels)

The results reported above were modified by adding the effect of the two level factor *area* with the following results:

1 *Asian partner and area effects*

	estimate	s.e.	t
Constant	0.504	0.305	1.65
Asian partner	-1.471	0.457	-3.22
Area	0.672	0.392	1.71

The components of deviance are as follows:

	d.f.	deviance
Asian partner	1	17.410
Area	1	2.909
Residual	137	166.383
Total	139	186.702

Comment: The Asian partnership effect is still negative and statistically significant. The 'area' effect is positive but not significant.

2 *The effect on average age*

	estimate	s.e.	t
Constant	0.112	0.361	0.31
Average age level 2	0.032	0.411	0.08
Average age level 3	-2.71	1.12	-2.42
Area	1.020	0.379	2.69

The components of deviance are as follows:

	d.f.	deviance
Age	2	12.703
Area	1	7.487
Residual	136	166.513

Comment: The 'area' and 'age' effects are jointly and separately statistically significant; the critical value of χ^2 is given above. The age effect is negative in the upper age range and the area effect is positive.

3 *The joint effect of area and working from a health centre*

	estimate	s.e.	t
Constant	-0.291	0.341	-0.86
Health centre	0.394	0.401	0.98
Area	0.994	0.372	2.67

The components of deviance are as follows:

	d.f.	deviance
Health centre	1	3.043
Area	1	7.307
Residual	137	176.352
Total	139	186.702

Comments: The area effect is statistically significant; the health centre effect is not. Critical value of χ^2 at 5% level is 3.84.

4 *The effect of RCGP membership and area together*

	estimate	s.e.	t
Constant	-0.713	0.311	-2.30
RCGP membership	1.431	0.381	3.75
Area	0.977	0.381	2.56

The components of deviance are as follows:

	d.f.	deviance
RCGP membership	1	17.560
Area	1	6.712
Residual	137	162.429
Total	139	186.702

Comment: Both RCGP membership and Area are statistically significant (at a level of significance less than 5%).

5 *The effect of income and area together*

	estimate	s.e.	t
Constant	-1.257	0.604	-2.08
Average net income level 2	0.746	0.724	1.03
Average net income level 3	1.445	0.683	2.11
Average net income level 4	1.243	0.725	1.71
Average net income level 5	2.374	0.774	3.07
Average net income level 6	2.52	1.23	2.05
Area	0.812	0.390	2.08

The components of deviance are as follows:

	d.f.	deviance
Average net income	5	19.410
Area	1	4.371
Residual	133	162.920
Total	139	186.702

Comment: Both average net income and Area are statistically significant (at a level of significance less than 5%).

6 *The effect of partnership size and area together*

	estimate	s.e.	t
Constant	-0.815	0.303	-2.69
Partnership size 4 - 5 partners	2.304	0.532	4.33
Partnership size > 5 partners	2.241	0.658	3.40
Area	0.878	0.405	2.17

The components of deviance are as follows:

	d.f.	deviance
Partnership size	2	36.511
Area	1	4.712
Residual	136	145.480
Total	139	186.702

Comment: As before, both partnership size (as defined) and area are statistically significant.

7 Adding area to the relationship derived by stepwise regression

	estimate	s.e.	t
Constant	0.003	0.450	0.01
Partnership size 4 - 5 partners	2.091	0.555	3.77
Partnership size > 5 partners	1.892	0.681	2.78
Asian partner	-1.378	0.518	-2.66
Average age level 2	-0.090	0.469	-0.19
Average age level 3	-2.13	1.14	-1.88
Area	0.488	0.450	1.08

	d.f.	deviance
Regression	6	53.3
Residual	133	133.4
Total	139	186.7

The components of deviance are as follows:

	d.f.	deviance
Partnership size	2	36.511
Asian partner	1	10.042
Average age	2	5.603
Area	1	1.147
Residual	133	133.400
Total	139	186.702

Comment: All effects except area are statistically significant.

Appendix 2 Informal views of family doctors

As well as more structured responses to questionnaires, family doctors made some informal comments.

In general, the doctors were more than happy to take part in the survey and give freely of their time. As one doctor put it typically:- "It is important that what GPs actually do should be known in more detail", and "I'm not very good at these type of things but will help if possible". Some, however, were more sceptical.

"I'm interested in patients, not economics"; "A lot of recent surveys have been used to discredit GPs"; "The results of the study might be used against us" and "most surveys are anti GP, and the object is to discredit them". It is to be hoped that the latter three doctors will be proved wrong about this survey. Others were sceptical about the Government:-

"The survey will end up on a minister's desk to be used against doctors", and "MPs never come into doctors' surgeries and talk to doctors about their problems".

Some were critical of the health service. "The quagmire of the NHS administration has nearly defeated me", and "Things are not necessarily any better now, in spite of modern technology".

Patients also came in for some criticism. "Patients should trust the doctor and listen to what he says"; "The health service has changed over the years. People now want pills with everything"; "More is being expected of doctors. This lady is 80 so in the natural course of things she will die, but now this is not acceptable" and "Doctors are continually under more pressure because of preventive medicine, a more knowledgeable public, with greater expectations and more elderly people".

One doctor felt that general practice "should be run as any other business should be". Another more cynically saw general practice in terms of "Lots of money for little work".

The variety of general practice

The interviewers themselves gave comments about the doctors they interviewed, and their premises. The selection below gives some indication of the variety of general practice.

1 *The doctors* Reception ranged from "practically a welcoming committee"; "The GP was friendly and welcoming"; "The doctor was very considerate and took time over each question"; "terrific"; "A very knowledgeable, energetic and informative GP, wish he were mine...", to the rather less enthusiastic. "I couldn't really decide whether he was being rude or whether it was just his manner"; "GP showed great lack of interest"; "After the initial question refused to go any further"; "An altogether fascinating and harrowing experience"; "Quite brisk and less welcoming than some", and "we rushed through it".

Sometimes there was initial nervousness or scepticism. "She was very interested but a bit nervous at first - I'm not sure what she was expecting"; "Not initially interested but ended up not being able to get away"; "He said he didn't want to spend a lot of time on the interview. I was there for one and a half hours".

2 *The premises* The premises ranged from "beautiful"; "old and beautiful and wildly impracticable"; "the surgery looked as though it had been arranged as a display room which could be used to demonstrate how a doctor's room should be organised"; "if only they could all be like this", and "slightly daunting for those used to seedier environments", to "...dying house plants and muddy carpets definitely detracted from my confidence in doctors"; "tatty", and finally "The room was thick with smoke and two full ashtrays were on the desk. No Smoking posters were displayed on two walls".

Index